VEGAN
MEAL PREP

EVERYDAY RECIPES

Kevin Smith

professional before attempting any techniques outlined in this book.

By reading this document, the reader agrees that under no circumstances is the author responsible for any losses, direct or indirect, which are incurred as a result of the use of information contained within this document, including, but not limited to, — errors, omissions, or inaccuracies.

Table of Contents

INTRODUCTION

The preparation of the meal. It is a subject that strikes in the heart of every new vegan, but do not fear, help is at hand!

Here, I will give you my best tips for preparing vegan meals, followed by a few simple recipes!

First of all, however, if you have decided to try to become vegan and are new to this lifestyle, welcome to a world of cooking that is full of flavor and beauty, and welcome to feel good knowing that what you eat contributes to making the world a kinder place.

We are fortunate that today we live in a world where there are many plant-based options (it seems that almost every day a different company/shop/restaurant launches new vegan products), making the preparation of vegan meals much more accessible. However, it can be daunting at first, and I understand that perfectly, so read on to find my best recipes on vegan meal preparation. I will have you prepared like a pro in no time!

Tips for preparing vegan meals

Cook in lots

Without doubt the most important advice of all, batch cooking is THE way to eliminate stress from preparing meals. Find some simple dishes that you like best (meals like soups, curries and salads are the best) and make large batches once a week. This way you'll have plenty of food for the week to come and don't have to worry about what to cook. You can also prepare large quantities of your favourite breakfasts and store them in the fridge for the night and then pick them up in the morning!

Plan your food

If you plan in advance what you will eat for breakfast, lunch and dinner every day at the beginning of the week, this eliminates a lot of stress from the kitchen and means you will never be hungry! Also, you'll never get home and you'll end up with empty cupboards because you've been shopping according to your plans.

Stick to your shopping list

As tempting as it is to shop without a list and think you'll remember everything you need for the week, believe me - you won't. After you've made your meal plan, write a shopping list and buy only these ingredients! You will avoid buying unnecessary items and reduce food waste.

Fill your fridge with the basic ingredients

Prepare a few simple items at the beginning of the week, such as (rice, millet, quinoa, etc.) to make sure you always have food on hand.

Go Simple

Keep things simple by preparing the dishes quickly and easily and save the more complicated meals for when you are a bit more experienced or have more time on your hands. Try to prepare delicious dishes from a single pot that produces many servings, such as hearty stews or curries. As you get used to eating from plants, you'll naturally want to branch out and try more challenging recipes, but make things as easy as possible for yourself to get started!

BREAKFAST

QUINOA BREAKFAST MEAL PREP

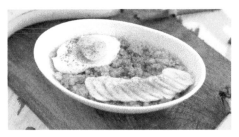

Prep Time: 5mints, Total Time: 20mints

Serving: 4

INGREDIENTS

- ➤ 1- cup quinoa
- ➤ 2- cups almond milk
- ➤ ½- teaspoon ground cinnamon
- ➤ ¼- teaspoon ground cardamom
- ➤ 2- tablespoons maple syrup
- ➤ 4- cups mixed berries
- ➤ 4- tablespoons sliced almonds

INSTRUCTIONS

- ✓ In a medium pot, be a part of the quinoa, almond milk, cinnamon, and cardamom.

- ✓ Heat to the factor of boiling, reduce warmth and stew for 15 or so mints until the quinoa is cooked through.

- ✓ Cool quinoa. Mix within the maple syrup, and partition into four compartments: ¾ cup cooked quinoa, 1 cup natural product, 1 tablespoon reduce almonds.

BANANA QUINOA BREAKFAST BARS

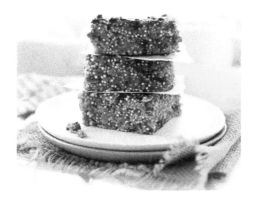

Prep Time: 20mints, Cook Time: 25mints, Total Time: 45mints

Serving: 9-12 bars

INGREDIENTS

- 1 cup rolled oats
- 1 cup uncooked white quinoa
- 1/2 tsp baking powder
- 1/2 tsp cinnamon
- Pinch of sea salt
- 3 large ripe bananas
- 2 tbsp ground flaxseed
- 3 tbsp natural peanut butter
- 1 tbsp coconut oil
- 2 tbsp pure maple syrup
- optional: 1/4-1/2 cup add-ins like chocolate chips, coconut, chopped dried fruit

- ✓ Preheat stove to 350 degrees F.

- ✓ Splash or oil a 9 x 9-inch heating dish with coconut oil

- ✓ In a huge bowl join moved oats, quinoa, preparing powder, cinnamon, and salt.

- ✓ Include bananas, flax, nutty spread, coconut oil, and maple syrup. Mix until well-consolidated.

- ✓ Sprinkle with discretionary include ins.

- ✓ Let batter sit for 10 mints to let flax ingest some fluid.

- ✓ Add batter to a heating dish and spread out uniformly.

- ✓ Heat for 25 mints or until edges are fresh and focus is cooked through.

- ✓ Let sit for 20 mints before cutting into 9-12 squares and permit to cool totally.

- ✓ Store in an impenetrable compartment for as long as 3 days or freeze for more.

SWEET POTATO AND BLACK BEAN BREAKFAST BURRITOS

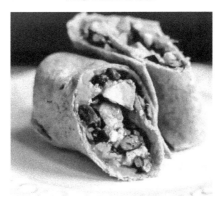

Prep Time: 10mints, Cook Time: 30mints, Total Time: 40mints

Serving: 3

INGREDIENTS

- 1 sweet potato
- 2 Tablespoons olive oil
- 1 teaspoon chili powder
- 1/2 teaspoon garlic powder
- 1/2 teaspoon paprika
- 1/2 teaspoon salt
- 1/4 teaspoon pepper
- 1/4 teaspoon cumin
- 1/4 teaspoon cayenne
- 1 can black beans
- 1 cup salsa
- 6 tortillas

INSTRUCTIONS

- ✓ Preheat the stove to 400 ranges.

- ✓ In a common bowl blend the sweet potato, olive oil, bean stew powder, garlic powder, paprika, salt, pepper, cumin, and cayenne. Spread out the candy potato mixture in an even layer onto a getting ready sheet. Heat for 25 mints

- ✓ At the factor, while the candy potatoes are completed, toss the dark beans onto the recent get a ready sheet and combine them.

- ✓ Amass the burrito by way of pouring half of cup sweet potato and darkish bean filling into the middle of a tortilla. Uniformly pour 1 Tablespoon of salsa over the candy potato mixture, and fold the tortilla into a burrito.

- ✓ When the whole thing of the burritos is gathered, warmth a vast skillet up over medium-high warmth

- ✓ At the factor, while the box is the recent spot each burrito into the skillet crease down.

- ✓ Darker for around 2 mints at that point turn the burritos over and darker for an additional 2 mints, Present with salsa and cilantro.

MAKE-AHEAD TOFU SCRAMBLE & BREAKFAST SWEET POTATOES

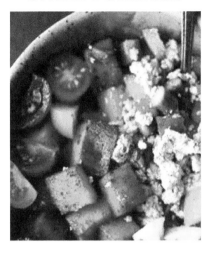

Prep Time: 15mints, Cook Time: 30mints, Total Time: 45mints

Serving: 3

INGREDIENTS

- 1.5 lbs sweet potato
- 1 tablespoon olive oil
- 2 teaspoons chili powder
- 1/2 teaspoon salt
- Tofu Scramble
- 1 block extra firm tofu

- 1/2 red onion
- 2 bell peppers
- 2 cups asparagus
- 1 teaspoon cumin
- 1 teaspoon ground coriander
- 1/2 teaspoon salt
- 1/4 teaspoon pepper

INSTRUCTIONS

- ✓ Preheat broiler to 425°F

- ✓ Toss sweet potatoes with olive oil, bean stew powder, and salt.

- ✓ Arrange on a preparing sheet, and heat for 15 mints. Work up and prepare for another 15-20 mints, until cooked through.

- ✓ While sweet potatoes heat, set up the tofu scramble: Mash the tofu with a potato masher until it is broken into little pieces.

- ✓ Warmth oil in a huge non-stick skillet.

- ✓ Include the onion, chime peppers and asparagus, and cook for 5 or so mints, until delicate.

- ✓ Include the cumin, ground coriander, salt, pepper, and tofu. Cook for 2-3 additional mints, until totally consolidated.

- ✓ To gather the morning meal bowls: Divide the tofu scramble and breakfast sweet potatoes among 6-8 holders. Store for as long as 4 days in the ice chest

✓ To serve Heat on medium in the microwave for 1 moment or until warmed through. Top with new cherry tomatoes, avocado, or potentially Greek yogurt.

ONE-BOWL MORNING GLORY MUFFINS

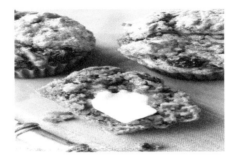

Prep Time: 15mints, Cook Time: 20mints, Total Time: 35mints

Serving: 1 dozen

INGREDIENTS

- 1 and 1/2 cups whole wheat flour
- 1/2 cup all-purpose flour
- 3/4 cup brown sugar
- 1 tablespoon baking powder
- 2 teaspoons baking soda
- 2 teaspoons ground cinnamon
- 1/2 teaspoon ground ginger
- 1/2 teaspoon salt
- 3/4 cup unsweetened applesauce
- 1/2 cup coconut oil
- 1 apple
- 1 tablespoon vanilla extract
- 2 cups grated carrot
- 1/2 cup raisins
- 1/2 cup flaked coconut
- 1/2 cup walnuts

INSTRUCTIONS

✓ Line a biscuit tin with paper liners and put them in a safe spot. Preheat broiler to 400 degrees

✓ In an enormous bowl includes the flours, sugar, heating powder, preparing pop, cinnamon, ginger, and salt; whisk well to consolidate. Include the fruit purée, oil, apple, and vanilla; whisk just until consolidated.

✓ Crease in the carrot, raisins, coconut, and pecans; mix until INGREDIENTS: are joined. Partition hitter equitably among arranged biscuit cups.

✓ Prepare at 400 degrees for 10 mints, at that point diminish the warmth to 350 degrees and heat for an extra 10 mints, or until a toothpick embedded in the inside confesses all.

✓ Cool biscuits in the search for gold mints before moving them to a wire rack. Serve warm, at room temperature, or chilled.

90-SECOND PUMPKIN PIE BREAKFAST QUINOA

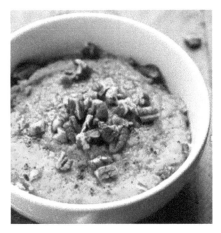

Prep Time: 2mints, Cook Time: 2mints, Total Time: 4mints

Servings: 1

INGREDIENTS

- 1/3 cup quinoa flakes
- 1/3 cup pumpkin puree
- 2 tablespoons maple sugar
- 1 1/4 cup plant-based milk
- 1/2 teaspoon cinnamon
- 1/4 teaspoon nutmeg
- 1/4 teaspoon ginger
- 1/4 teaspoon vanilla bean powder
- Pecans + additional maple sugar for topping optional

INSTRUCTIONS

- ✓ Consolidate the quinoa drops, pumpkin, maple sugar and milk in a little pot.

- ✓ Heat to the point of boiling at that point diminish to stew, mixing continually until thickened, around 90 seconds. Mix in flavors.

- ✓ Move to a bowl, and top with walnuts and maple sugar if utilizing.

MEGAN CARROT CAKE QUINOA BREAKFAST BARS

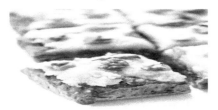

Prep Time: 10mints, Cook Time: 25mints, Total Time: 35mints

Servings: 16 bars

INGREDIENTS

- 1 flax egg 1½ tablespoons flaxseed meal + 3 tablespoons water
- 1 cup cooked chickpeas
- ½ cup mashed banana about 1 large banana
- ½ cup unsweetened applesauce
- ¾ cup quinoa flour
- ½ cup of coconut sugar
- 1 teaspoon ground cinnamon
- ½ teaspoon ground nutmeg
- ½ teaspoon ground vanilla bean
- ½ teaspoon baking soda
- Pinch of salt
- ¼ cup hemp hearts
- ½ cup grated carrots
- ¼ cup chopped walnuts
- Coconut Buttercream Frosting optional

✓ Preheat the stove to 350°F. Oil and line an 8x8 heating dish with fabric and put it in a secure spot.

✓ Whisk together the flaxseed dinner and water in a bit bowl. Put in a secure spot for 5 mints.

✓ In the interim, blend the chickpeas, banana, and fruit purée in a nourishment processor till totally easy.

✓ In a massive blending bowl, whisk together the dry INGREDIENTS:, keeping the hemp hearts, carrot, and pecans. Empty the chickpea puree into the bowl along the flax egg and blend to consolidate.

✓ Overlay in the hemp hearts, ground carrot, and pecans.

✓ Dump the hitter into the readied skillet. Prepare at the center rack for 22 - 26 mints till a toothpick embedded into the inner tells the fact.

✓ Give cool get entry to the look for gold - 15 mints, at that point move to a twine rack and cool completely before icing and cutting.

✓ Cut into 12 - sixteen bars. Store in a hermetically sealed compartment for 2 - 3 days

OATMEAL PEANUT BUTTER BREAKFAST COOKIES

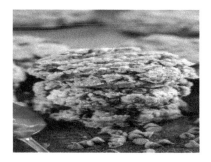

Prep Time: 10mints, Cook Time: 15mints, Total Time: 25mints

Serving: 4

INGREDIENTS

- 1 ¼ cups rolled oats
- ¼ cup oat flour
- ½ cup almond flour
- ½ teaspoon baking soda
- ½ teaspoon fine kosher or sea salt
- ½ cup Santa Cruz Organic creamy dark roasted peanut butter
- ½ cup Santa Cruz Organic apple sauce
- 3 tablespoons maple syrup
- 3 tablespoons coconut oil
- 1 teaspoon vanilla extract
- 2 tablespoons flax meal
- 2 tablespoons Santa Cruz Organic fruit spread
- 1/3 cup dark chocolate chips

- ✓ Preheat the broiler to 350 stages F. Line a treat sheet with fabric paper or a silicone tangle.

- ✓ In an average bowl, speed collectively the oats, oat flour, almond flour, making ready pop, and salt.

- ✓ In every other littler bowl, whisk together the nutty spread, fruit purée, maple syrup, coconut oil, vanilla concentrate, and flax supper till clean.

- ✓ Mix the moist INGREDIENTS: into the dry INGREDIENTS: till consolidated.

- ✓ Drop tablespoon-sized bundles of aggregate onto the handled sheet and stage right into a treat form.

- ✓ On the occasion that created the nutty spread and jam thumbprint treats, utilize a lubed teaspoon to make an area.

- ✓ Fill the areas with herbal products unfold. Heat treats 12-15 mints, until great

PEACH PIE BREAKFAST PARFAITS

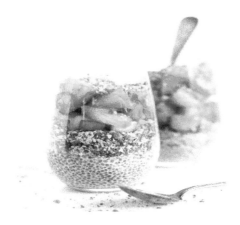

Prep Time: 10mints, Cook Time: 5mints, Total Time: 2hrs 15mints

Servings: 2

- ¼- cup chia seeds
- 1- tablespoon pure maple syrup
- 1- cup plant milk
- 2/3- cups rolled oats gluten-free
- 1/3- cup raw pecans
- 5 – 6- Medjool dates depending on the size
- 2- teaspoons cinnamon
- 3- medium peaches

- ✓ Make the chia pudding: join the chia seeds, syrup and almond milk in a bowl or the huge mason container. Combine until fused, at that point refrigerate to set for in any event 2 hours.

- ✓ Make the disintegrate: toast oats and walnuts in a dry skillet over medium warmth until brilliant darker, around 5 mints. When toasted, move to a nourishment processor alongside dates and 1 teaspoon of cinnamon. The procedure to frame the surface of coarse sand.

- ✓ Make the peaches: cut the peaches down the middle, dispose of the pit, and cleaving into reduced down pieces. Add to a bowl with the staying 1 teaspoon of cinnamon and toss to join.

- ✓ Gather the parfaits: separate the chia pudding equitably among two stemless wine glasses or mason containers.

- ✓ Include a layer of the disintegrate, at that point isolate peaches equitably and place them over the disintegrate. Sprinkle with a bit of disintegrate beating and enjoy it!

ULTIMATE NO-BAKE BREAKFAST COOKIE BITES

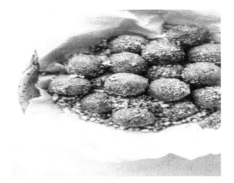

Prep Time: 20mints, Cooking Time: 30mints, Total Time: 50mints

Serving: 4

INGREDIENTS

- 1/3- cup ground oats
- 1- cup almond flour
- ¼ to 1/3- cup peanut flour
- 2- tbsp chia
- ¼- c natural nut butter
- 1- tbsp cinnamon
- ¼- cup maple syrup
- ½- tsp vanilla
- 1- tbsp molasses
- dark chocolate shavings
- extra flour/cinnamon to sprinkle on top

- ✓ Finely pound 1/2 cup entire moved oats in a nourishment processor or blender, at that point move into a blending bowl. This should make around 1/3 cup ground oats. You can likewise simply utilize oat flour.

- ✓ Include your almond flour, nut flour or protein powder, cinnamon, chia or flaxseed, and almond spread.

- ✓ Mix INGREDIENTS: all together. Include your maple syrup, molasses, and vanilla at that point blend again with hands. In the event that you are including nuts, do as such here. Only 1 tbsp.

- ✓ You may need to include more maple syrup or almond margarine if the hitter gets the opportunity to dry.

- ✓ Fold into 1-1.5 inch balls. At that point roll each ball in a couple of squashed nuts and spot it on a heating sheet or another enormous holder with material paper underneath.

- ✓ Let them freeze for 20-30 mints at that point move into a Ziploc pack.

- ✓ Residue with extra cinnamon and nut flour whenever wanted. keep in an ice chest or cooler for as long as about a month and a half

THE ULTIMATE VEGAN BREAKFAST BURRITO

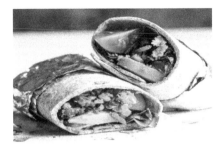

Prep Time: 20mints, Cook Time: 20mints, Total Time: 40mints

Servings: 3

- Other INGREDIENTS:
- 4 wholewheat wraps
- 1 Green Bell Pepper
- 7-8 Cherry Tomatoes
- 1 Avocado
- Fresh Spinach
- Salsa
- Scrambled Chickpeas
- 400g chickpeas
- 1/4 tsp Garlic Powder
- 1/2 tsp Ground Cumin
- 1/4 tsp Chilli Powder
- 1/4 tsp Smoked Paprika
- 1 pinch Ground Turmeric
- Seitan "Bacon"
- 3.5oz Seitan
- 1/2 tsp Chilli Powder
- 1/4 tsp Smoked Paprika
- 1/4 tsp Ground Cumin
- salt and pepper

INSTRUCTIONS

- ✓ Preheat the range to one hundred eighty°C. Cut the green chime pepper into strips and spot on a degree heating sheet along with the cherry tomatoes. Broil for 20-25 mints till sensitive and a touch singed.

- ✓ In the period in-between, pound the chickpeas utilizing the rear of a fork, or hastily beat them inside the nourishment processor until they may be stout. Blend in with each one of the flavors and mix so everything is included.

- ✓ Utilize a vegetable peeler to reduce the seitan into flimsy strips, at that point combination in with each one of the flavors and toss so each one of the pieces is covered.

- ✓ Warmth 1 tbsp olive oil in a large skillet. Spot the chickpeas on one facet, and the seitan on the opposite aspect and prepare dinner for 5-10 mints until definitely warm right thru. Mix the 2 sides regularly.

- ✓ Collect the burritos with the seitan, chickpeas, some cooked peppers and tomatoes, new spinach, avocado, and salsa. Serve right away.

EASY VEGAN BREAKFAST TACOS

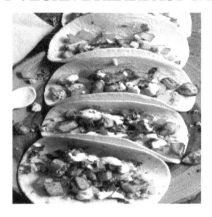

Prep Time: 15mints, Cook Time: 15mints, Total Time: 30mints

Serving: 3

INGREDIENTS

- TACOS:
- 8 ounces firm tofu
- 1 cup cooked black beans
- 1/4 red onion
- 1 cup fresh cilantro
- 1 ripe avocado
- 1/2 cup salsa
- 1 medium lime
- 1/4 cup pomegranate arils
- 6 whole corn tortillas
- TOFU SEASONING:
- 3/4 tsp garlic powder
- 1/2 tsp chili powder
- 1 tsp cumin
- 1/8 tsp sea salt
- 1 Tbsp salsa
- 1 Tbsp water

- ✓ Envelop tofu by a perfect, spongy towel and see something massive on pinnacle, as an example, a cast-iron skillet, while getting ready garnishes.

- ✓ Cook dark beans in a bit pan over medium warmth until bubbly. At that factor decrease warmth to stew and keep. On the off threat that unsalted/unseasoned, include a touch of salt, cumin, bean stew powder, and garlic powder.

- ✓ Include dry tofu flavors + salsa to a touch bowl and add sufficient water to make a pourable sauce. Put in a secure spot.

- ✓ Warmth a massive skillet over medium warm temperature and unwrap tofu. Utilize a fork to crumble.

- ✓ When the dish is hot, include 1-2 Tbsp oil of selection and the tofu. Pan-fried meals for four-five mints to dark-colored. At that point add flavoring and toss to cowl. Keep cooking until seared and aromatic - around 5-10 mints - mixing frequently. Put in a secure spot.

- ✓ To serve, heat tortillas within the microwave enveloped by way of a soggy paper towel or in a 250-diploma F. Top tortillas with tofu scramble, dark beans, onion, avocado, cilantro, salsa, crisp lime juice, and pomegranate arils.

- ✓ Serve quick with the best breakfast potatoes or organic product.

VEGAN FRIENDLY CINNAMON VANILLA PROTEIN BREAKFAST BITES

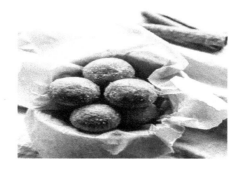

Prep Time: 12min, Total Time: 12min

Serving: 16-18 bites

INGREDIENTS

- ➤ 3/4 cup of gluten-free rolled oats
- ➤ 1/4 cup Vanilla Protein Powder
- ➤ 1/2 cup almond flour
- ➤ 1 heaping tablespoon ground Cinnamon
- ➤ 1/4 to 1/3 cup nut butter or sunflower seed butter
- ➤ 1/2 tsp to 1 tsp Vanilla extract
- ➤ 1/4 to 1/3 cup maple syrup

INSTRUCTIONS

- ✓ Crush your oats or grain in a nourishment processor and move it into a blending bowl. This is discretionary. You can keep them entire too and change the expansion of nectar.

- ✓ Include your almond supper, protein powder, cinnamon, and nut margarine. Mix INGREDIENTS: all together.
- ✓ Include your nectar and vanilla at that point blend again well in with hands.
- ✓ You may need to include progressively nectar or nut margarine if the hitter gets the chance to dry.
- ✓ Fold into 1-1.5 inch balls and spot on a treat plate or plastic product with material paper underneath.
- ✓ Let them freeze for 20-30 mints at that point move into a Ziploc sack.
- ✓ Residue with extra cinnamon and vanilla protein whenever wanted
- ✓ Keep in the ice chest or cooler for as long as about a month and a half.

BREAKFAST GRAIN SALAD WITH BLUEBERRIES, HAZELNUTS & LEMON

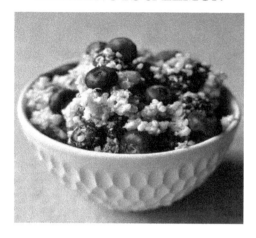

Prep Time: 15mints, Cooking Time: 30mints, Total Time: 45mints

Serving: 8

INGREDIENTS

- 1 cup steel-cut oats
- 1 cup dry golden quinoa
- 1/2 cup dry millet
- 3 tablespoons olive oil
- 1-inch fresh ginger
- 2 large lemons, zest and juice
- 1/2 cup maple syrup
- 1 cup Greek yogurt
- 1/4 teaspoon nutmeg
- 2 cups hazelnuts
- 2 cups blueberries or mixed berries

INSTRUCTIONS

- ✓ Blend the oats, quinoa, and millet in a fine-work strainer and wash for about a moment under running water. Put in a safe spot.

- ✓ Include the washed grains and cook for 2 to 3 mints or until they start smelling toasted.

- ✓ Pour 4 1/2 cups water and mix in 3/4 teaspoon salt, the ginger coins, and the get-up-and-go of 1 lemon. Bring to a bubble, spread, turn down the warmth, and stew for 20 mints.

- ✓ Mood killer the warmth and let sit for 5 mints, at that point evacuate the cover and lighten with a fork.

- ✓ Remove the ginger. Spread hot grains on an enormous preparing sheet and let cool for in any event thirty mints.

- ✓ Spoon the cooled grains into an enormous bowl. Mix in the pizzazz of the subsequent lemon.

- ✓ In a medium bowl, whisk the staying 2 tablespoons olive oil with the juice of the two lemons until emulsified. Speed in the maple syrup, yogurt, and nutmeg. Empty this into the grains and mix until well-covered.

✓ Mix in the toasted hazelnuts and blueberries. Taste and season with extra salt, if vital

✓ Refrigerate medium-term; the kinds of this truly met up medium-term in the refrigerator.

LEMON BLUEBERRY – HEALTHY MAKE-AHEAD BREAKFAST COOKIES

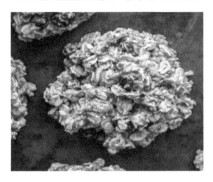

Prep Time: 10mints, Cook Time: 15mints, Total Time: 25mints

Serving: 12

INGREDIENTS

- 2 1/2 cups old fashioned oats
- 3/4 cups flour
- 1/4 cup coconut sugar
- 1 teaspoon baking powder
- 1/2 teaspoon ground cinnamon
- 1/8 teaspoon salt
- 1/2 cup + 1 tablespoon non-dairy milk
- 1/4 cup maple syrup
- 1 flax egg
- 1 teaspoon vanilla extract
- 1 1/2 teaspoons lemon zest
- 2 teaspoons lemon juice
- 1/2 cup dried blueberries

INSTRUCTIONS

✓ Pre-warmth stove to 350 stages F and line a big getting ready sheet with material paper.

✓ Add every dry solving to a large bowl and mix. Next, include every outstanding ingredient and blend again until the whole thing is consolidated.

✓ Utilize a 1/four cup scoop to scoop the hitter onto the material paper. Pat the tops down a little and warmth treat for 15-17 mints, till firm and cooked via. Let cool on a twine rack before ingesting.

VEGAN BREAKFAST MUFFINS

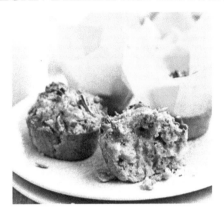

Prep Time: 25mints, Cook Time: 25mints, Total Time: 50mints

Serving: 4

INGREDIENTS

- 150g muesli mix
- 50g light brown soft sugar
- 160g plain flour
- 1 tsp baking powder
- Baking powder
- 250ml sweetened soy milk
- 1 apple
- Apples
- 2 tbsp grapeseed oil
- 3 tbsp nut butter
- 4 tbsp demerara sugar
- 50g pecans
- Pecan nuts

✓ Warmth the range to 200C/180C fan/gasoline 6. Line a biscuit tin with cases. Blend 100g muesli in with the light-darkish colored sugar, flour, and heating powder in a bowl. Join the milk, apple, oil and 2 tbsp nut unfold in a field, at that factor blend into the dry combo.

✓ Partition similarly among the cases. Blend the rest of the muesli in with the demerara sugar, final nut margarine, and the walnuts, and spoon over the biscuits.

✓ Prepare for 25-30 mints or until the biscuits are risen and tremendous. Will maintain for a few days in a water/air proof holder or freeze for one month. Invigorate inside the range before serving.

MAKE-AHEAD DETOX QUINOA BREAKFAST BOWLS

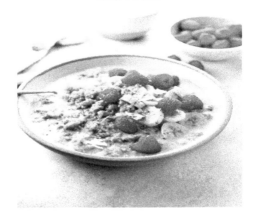

Prep Time: 25mints, Cook Time: 1minute, Total Time: 25mints

Servings: 6

- Quinoa:
- 1 ½- cups quinoa
- 15- ounce coconut milk or milk of choice
- 1 1/2 cups water
- 1 teaspoon ground cinnamon
- 1/4 cup pure maple syrup
- 2 teaspoons vanilla extract
- 1/4 teaspoon salt
- Optional toppings:
- Fresh fruit
- Coconut flakes
- Hemp hearts
- Non-dairy milk

✓ Channel the splashed quinoa and rince well. Spot the quinoa in the bowl of your Instant Pot, alongside the coconut milk, water, cinnamon, maple syrup, vanilla, and salt. Seal the cover with the vent shut, and press the catch for the "rice" setting.

✓ Enable the strain to normally discharge, around 10 mints, at that point open the vent at the top and remove the cover.

✓ Separation the quinoa into 6 individual compartments with tops, and store them in the ice chest until prepared to serve.

✓ At the point when you're prepared to have breakfast, top one presenting with non-dairy milk, crisp organic product, coconut pieces, hemp hearts, and some other garnishes you like.

MAKE-AHEAD BREAKFAST JARS

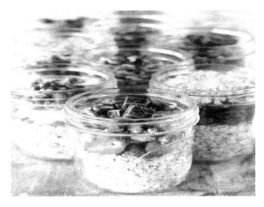

Prep Time: 10mints, Cook Time: 8hours, Total Time: 8hrs 10mints

Serving: 4

INGREDIENTS

- ➢ 1 serving smoothie, chia pudding
- ➢ 1/3 cup favorite toppings
- ➢ 1 wide-mouth pint canning jar and lid
- ➢ 1 empty plastic applesauce container

INSTRUCTIONS

- ✓ Fill the container with your elements for chia pudding or medium-term cereal, or a readied smoothie. In the case of freezing smoothies, make certain to leave space for extension while freezing with the goal that the container doesn't break.

✓ Fill the vacant fruit purée compartment with your garnishes. Spot the container top-side-down to cover the garnishes in the fruit purée holder. Cautiously turn the garnishes, secured with the cover, onto the filled container.

✓ Utilize the jostling to seal. Refrigerate chia pudding and oats medium-term. Freeze smoothies.

✓ Chia pudding ought to be eaten cold. Medium-term oats can be warmed in the microwave, yet evacuate the INGREDIENTS: first! Remove the smoothie from the cooler 1-2 hours before eating to give it an opportunity to defrost a piece.

VEGAN BREAKFAST TACOS NO TOFU!

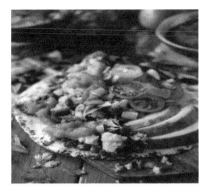

Prep Time: 15mints, Cook Time: 15mints, Total Time: 30mints.

Serving: 8

- 8- small corn tortillas
- 1- bell pepper
- 1- small red onion
- 1- ripe avocado
- ½- lime
- 1½- T vegetable oil
- 2- cans pinto beans
- ⅔- C vegetable stock, bean cooking liquid, or water
- 4- C baby spinach or other mild greens
- 2- T roughly chopped cilantro
- Salt
- Ground black pepper
- To serve: roughly chopped cilantro, salsa

✓ Warmth the tortillas. Roast them over a low fuel fire until obscured in simplest a couple of spots on the 2 facets, or, warmth a medium solid iron or nonstick skillet over medium-high warm temperature.

✓ Warm tortillas for approximately a second on each facet inside the dry dish, at that factor move to an extensive little bit of foil and crease over to hold heat. Move the package deal of tortillas to the microwave or a low range while you installation the filling.

✓ Cleave the ringer pepper and onion. Cut the avocado and toss with juice from a fourth of lime further to a hint of salt.

✓ At the factor when you're completed warming the tortillas, heat oil over medium-high within the skillet until very hot. Include the peppers and onions and mix rarely, till sautéed and modestly sensitive. Include beans, stock, and ½ teaspoon salt. Heat to the factor of boiling, at that factor stew round 5 mints, pounding a part of the beans in opposition to the bottom of the container with a spoon or spatula

✓ At the point while a tad of fluid stays, decrease warmth to medium-low, consist of the spinach, and blend. Cook a couple of mints, till spinach is withered, at that point encompass juice from a fourth of the lime, the cilantro, and salt and pepper to flavor.

✓ To serve, top every tortilla with a scoop of beans, more than one cuts of avocado, and some salsa. Sprinkle with cilantro, at that point overlap into equal components or roll.

VEGAN PEANUT BUTTER CHOCOLATE OVERNIGHT OATS

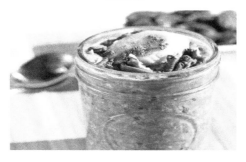

Prep Time: 5mints, Total Time: 5mints

Serving: 4

INGREDIENTS

- Peanut Butter Layer
- 1 cup quick-cooking oats
- 1.25 cups Silk Unsweetened Vanilla Almondmilk
- 2 teaspoons chia seeds
- 1 tablespoon honey
- 2 teaspoons ground flax seed
- 2 tablespoons all-natural peanut butter
- pinch of salt
- Chocolate Later
- 1 cup quick-cooking oats
- 1.5 cups Silk Unsweetened Vanilla Almondmilk
- 2 teaspoons chia seeds
- 1 tablespoon maple syrup
- 2 teaspoons ground flax seed

- ➢ 3 tablespoons cocoa powder
- ➢ pinch of salt
- ➢ Optional toppings
- ➢ all natural peanut butter
- ➢ mini chocolate chips

- ✓ **For the Peanut Butter Layer:** Spot all INGREDIENTS: into a glass Tupperware and blend. Spot in the fridge for in any event 2 hours or medium-term.

- ✓ For the Chocolate Layer:

- ✓ Spot all INGREDIENTS: into a glass Tupperware and blend. Spot in the fridge for in any event 2 hours or medium-term.

- ✓ **For the Peanut Butter Cup Overnight Oats:** In a container, layer the nutty spread and chocolate medium-term oat blend. Top with all characteristic nutty spread and a couple of chocolate chips.

PEANUT BUTTER BANANA OVERNIGHT OATS

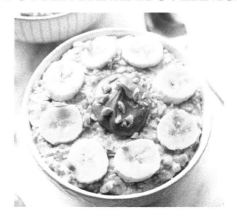

Prep Time: 5mints, Cook Time: 5mints, Total Time: 10mints

Serves: 1

INGREDIENTS

- ➢ 1 cup almond milk
- ➢ ½ cup gluten-free certified old fashioned oats
- ➢ 1 banana
- ➢ ¼ teaspoon cinnamon
- ➢ 1 teaspoon coconut sugar
- ➢ 1 tablespoon peanut butter
- ➢ optional: coconut flakes, chopped nuts, chia seeds

INSTRUCTIONS

- ✓ Combine all the INGREDIENTS: in a receptacle, without bananas.

- ✓ You can encompass the bananas at the pinnacle or mixture in thereafter.

- ✓ Spot inside the cooler medium-time period.

- ✓ The following morning, remove and eat inside the field or spot in a pot over medium-high warm temperature to warm the oats, or inside the microwave to heat if a microwave-secure box for around 45 seconds.

- ✓ Top with your selected garnishes - pecans, chia seeds, regularly nutty spread, and extra coconut sugar.

- ✓ Enjoy!

SCRAMBLED TOFU BREAKFAST TACOS

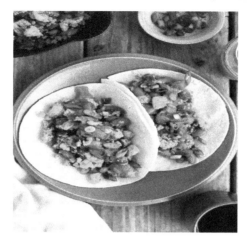

Prep Time: 5mints, Cook Time: 10mints, Total Time: 15mints

Serving: 4

INGREDIENTS

- 1 teaspoon olive oil
- 1 red pepper
- 1 clove garlic
- 1 package super firm Nasoya Tofu
- 1/4 teaspoon ground turmeric
- 1/4 teaspoon cumin
- 1/4 teaspoon salt
- Freshly ground black pepper
- 8 corn tortillas
- 1 avocado
- 1/2 cup grape tomatoes
- Optional: 1/2 cup goat cheese crumbles
- Optional: Hot sauce & cilantro, to garnish

- ✓ Add oil to an enormous skillet and spot over medium warmth. Include diced red pepper and garlic and saute for 2 mints.

- ✓ Next, disintegrate the tofu with your hands and add to the container. Sprinkle in flavors and salt and pepper. Cook for 5 mints; blending much of the time. Taste and include progressively salt and pepper are essential.

- ✓ Gap tofu scramble between tortillas, at that point top with avocado, tomatoes, and goat cheddar. Enhancement with your preferred hot sauce and cilantro. Enjoy! Makes 8 tacos all out. Serving size: 2 tacos for each individual

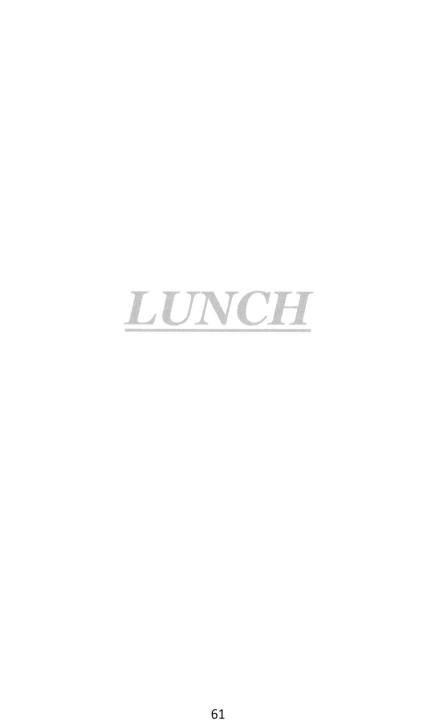

LUNCH

CAULIFLOWER CASHEW LUNCH BOWLS

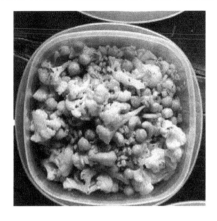

Prep Time: 15mints, Cook Time: 45mints, Total Time: 1hr

Servings: 5

INGREDIENTS

- ➤ Vinaigrette
- ➤ 1/4 cup olive oil
- ➤ 1/4 cup white wine vinegar
- ➤ 2 tablespoons honey
- ➤ 1/2 teaspoon dijon
- ➤ 2 teaspoons grated ginger using the fine art of the box grater

- ➤ Salad
- ➤ 2/3 cup uncooked pearl barley
- ➤ 1 head cauliflower
- ➤ 1 tablespoon olive oil
- ➤ 1/2 cup cashews
- ➤ 1/4 cup red onion
- ➤ 1 can chickpeas
- ➤ salt and pepper

- ✓ Cook pearl grain as per bundle bearings

- ✓ Pre-heat stove to 400°F.

- ✓ Toss the cauliflower with the olive oil in a huge bowl and sprinkle with salt and pepper.

- ✓ Spread cauliflower on a huge preparing sheet.

- ✓ Broil cauliflower, turning every so often, for 30-45 mints, until delicate and brilliant in places.

- ✓ Add the cashews to the stove for the last 5 or so mints, or until delicately brilliant.

- ✓ Shake together all vinaigrette INGREDIENTS:.

- ✓ Prepare all plate of mixed greens INGREDIENTS: together, separate into 5 sealable lunch holders, and store refrigerated until you're prepared to eat.

MAKE-AHEAD ENCHILADA LUNCH BOWLS

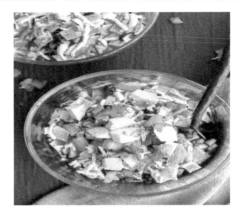

Prep Time: 20mints, Cook Time: 30mints, Total Time: 50mints

Serving: 4

INGREDIENTS

- 1 red pepper
- 1 small zucchini
- 1 small summer squash
- 1/2 small onion
- 1 cup corn kernels
- 15- ounce black beans
- 6 corn tortillas
- 19- oz enchilada sauce
- 1 cup shredded cheese
- 1 teaspoon olive oil
- 1 teaspoon ground cumin
- 1 teaspoon paprika
- 1 teaspoon garlic powder
- 3/4 teaspoon salt
- 1/4 teaspoon black pepper

- ✓ Preheat broiler to 375 F. Warmth a huge skillet over medium warmth and include the olive oil and every one of the veggies. Cook veggies until relaxed, 5-7 mints. Next, include the dark beans and every one of the flavors. Mix and cook for an additional 2 mints.

- ✓ Collect lunch bowls in a little stove safe pyrex dish. For each bowl, add 2 tablespoons enchilada sauce to the base and afterward top with 1/2 cup veggie blend, 1/4 cup cleaved corn tortillas, 1-2 tablespoons cheddar and afterward 2 additional tablespoons enchilada sauce.

- ✓ Rehash again finishing with a layer of cheddar on top. It's least demanding in the event that you fill every one of the dishes simultaneously.

- ✓ Spot bowls on an enormous preparing sheet and stick in the stove until cheddar is dissolved and enchiladas are bubbly around 20 mints. Remove from broiler and let cool before putting covers on top and refrigerating until required.

MISO GLAZED SWEET POTATO BOWLS

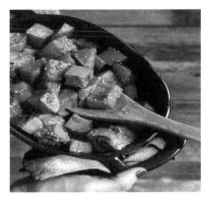

Prep Time: 15mints, Cook Time: 45mints, Total Time: 1hour

Serving: 4 bowls

INGREDIENTS

- 2 medium sweet potatoes
- 1 and 1/2 cups uncooked farro
- 1 teaspoon ground turmeric
- 3 tablespoons white miso
- 2 tablespoons low sodium tamari
- 1 tablespoon rice wine vinegar
- 2 tablespoons pure maple syrup
- 1 tablespoon extra virgin olive oil
- 1 onion
- 5 cups chopped kale
- 8 ounces mushrooms
- 1 teaspoon garlic powder
- Avocado and tahini sauce

- ✓ Preheat the broiler to 425°F at that point line a getting ready sheet with fabric paper. Organize the diced sweet potato on top and heat within the range for around 20-25 mints, till delicate, mixing partially via.

- ✓ In a touch pot, warmth three cups water to the point of boiling. Include the farro and cook dinner for round 20 mints, till delicate. When everything of the water has ate up, add the turmeric and mix to enroll in.

- ✓ In a massive pot, heat the olive oil over medium warmth. Include the onion and prepare dinner for 3 mints.

- ✓ Include the mushrooms, sprinkle with salt and pepper and garlic powder, at that factor prepare dinner for round 5 mints, till the mushrooms discharge their fluid. In end, consist of the kale and cook dinner for round 5-7 mints, until withered.

- ✓ In a massive bowl. Whisk collectively the miso, tamari, rice wine vinegar, unadulterated maple syrup, and 1/4 cup water till easy. Add the candy potatoes to the bowl and toss till equitably protected.

- ✓ Organize the candy potatoes in isolates bowls with the farro and the kale/mushroom mixture. Top with avocado and tahini sauce, and admire!

VEGAN MOROCCAN CHICKPEA SKILLET

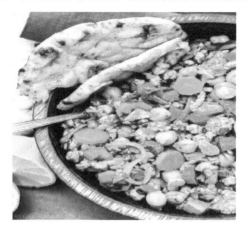

Prep Time: 15mints, Cook Time: 30mints, Total Time: 45mints

Serving: 4

INGREDIENTS

- 15 oz chickpeas
- 19 oz can of diced tomatoes
- 1 bell pepper
- 2 cups sweet potato
- 1 onion
- 1 ½- tsp Homemade Moroccan Spice Blend
- 1/4 teaspoon salt
- To serve:
- 1/2 lemon
- Parsley

- ✓ Add all INGREDIENTS: to a huge skillet and work up. Spread and stew for 30 mints or until sweet potatoes are cooked through, working up once in a while.

- ✓ On the off chance that you see the skillet getting dry, include 1/2 cup water or stock and spread.

- ✓ To collect ahead and freeze

- ✓ Join all INGREDIENTS: in a decent quality gallon-sized cooler sack. Crush out however much air as could reasonably be expected and freeze level for as long as 3 months.

- ✓ Defrost totally before cooking in the skillet as coordinated previously. Start checking for doneness at 15 mints.

VEGAN ROASTED VEGETABLE MEAL PREP

TURMERIC TAHINI SAUCE

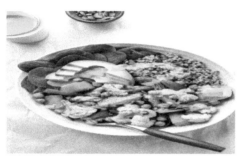

Prep Time: 20mints, Cook Time: 30mints, Total Time: 50mints

Serving: 5

INGREDIENTS

- 3/- cup uncooked quinoa
- 2- cups butternut squash
- 2- cups broccoli
- 2- cups cauliflower
- 1- tablespoon olive oil
- Salt & pepper
- 15- oz chickpeas
- Turmeric Tahini Sauce
- ¼- cup tahini
- 1 ½- tablespoons lemon juice
- 1 ½- tablespoons maple syrup
- 2- tablespoons water
- ¼- teaspoon cumin
- ¼- teaspoon ground coriander
- ¼- teaspoon garlic powder
- ½- teaspoon turmeric
- 1/8- teaspoon salt

- ✓ Cook quinoa as indicated by bundle headings. Separation out into four 2-cup limit dinner prep compartments

- ✓ Warmth broiler to 425°F.

- ✓ Toss the butternut squash, broccoli, and cauliflower in olive oil. Organize on an enormous preparing sheet and sprinkle with salt and pepper.

- ✓ Broil vegetables for 20-30 mints, until delicate and cooked through. Butternut squash may take somewhat longer than the broccoli and cauliflower.

- ✓ Partition simmered veggies and jar of chickpeas between the four dinner prep holders.

- ✓ Shake together all elements for the turmeric tahini sauce and bit out into four ingredient holders.

VEGAN BANANA CHOCOLATE DONUTS

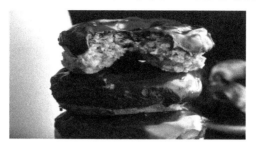

Prep Time: 5mints, Cook Time: 13mints, Total Time: 18mints

Servings: 6 donuts

INGREDIENTS

- 1 banana
- 1/2 cup almond milk
- 2 tablespoons almond oil
- 2 tablespoons peanut butter
- 1 teaspoon apple cider vinegar
- 1 teaspoon vanilla extract
- 1 1/4 cups quick-cooking oats
- 1/2 cup almond flour
- 1/2 cup coconut sugar
- 1/4 cup cacao powder
- 1/2 teaspoon baking soda
- 1/4 teaspoon sea salt
- 1/3 cup vegan dark chocolate chips
- 1/2 cup organic powdered sugar
- 2 tablespoons peanut butter powder
- 2 - 4 teaspoons almond milk

INSTRUCTIONS

✓ Preheat the stove to 350°F. Oil a doughnut skillet and put it in a safe spot.

✓ In the request recorded, add all INGREDIENTS: to a blender and mix on high until smooth. The blend will be thick!

✓ Include your chocolate chips into the blender and crease into the batter with a spatula.

✓ Spoon the hitter into the readied doughnut skillet, filling every right to the top. Prepare for 13 - 14 mints until the doughnuts are springy to the touch. Remove from the broiler and let cool in the search for gold at least 15 mints.

✓ Once cooled, flip the doughnuts out onto a wire rack and cool totally.

✓ On the off chance that you need to make the coating, whisk together the powdered sugar, powdered nutty spread, and almond milk and shower over the doughnuts. Enjoy promptly or store at room temperature in a water/air proof compartment for 2 days.

NO-BAKE SNACK BARS

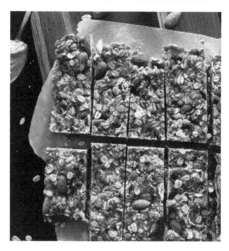

Prep Time: 15mints, Cooking Time: 2hrs, Total Time: 2hrs 15mints

Servings: 16

INGREDIENTS

- ➢ 1/4 cup coconut oil
- ➢ 2/3 cup peanut butter
- ➢ 1/2 cup maple syrup
- ➢ 1/2 teaspoon cinnamon
- ➢ 1 cup rolled oats
- ➢ 1 cup Rice Krispies
- ➢ 1/2 cup ground flaxseed
- ➢ 1/2 cup chocolate chips
- ➢ 1/4 cup chia seeds

INSTRUCTIONS

✓ Liquefy coconut oil in an enormous bowl.

✓ Mix in the nutty spread, maple syrup, and cinnamon until smooth.

✓ Mix in the oats, Rice Krispies, flax and chocolate chips.

✓ Line an 8 x 8-inch container with the material. Press the blend into the container until smooth over the top.

✓ Refrigerate for in any event 2 hours, at that point cut into bars and segment out for the week.

VEGAN THE BEST KALE CHIPS

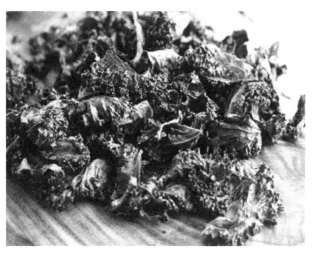

Prep Time: 5mints, Cook Time: 8mints, Total Time: 13mints

Serving: 2

INGREDIENTS

- 2 large stalks kale
- 1 TBS avocado oil
- 1 1/2 TBS nutritional yeast
- 1/2 tsp garlic powder
- 1/4 tsp cumin
- 1/4 tsp chili powder
- 1/8 tsp cayenne
- 1/4 tsp pink salt

INSTRUCTIONS

- ✓ Preheat stove to 300°F. Oil an enormous heating sheet and put it in a safe spot.

- ✓ Cautiously remove leaves from the stalk of the kale. You can either pull the leaves or remove them from the stalk. Tear or cut kale into huge pieces, at that point wash and dry kale in a serving of mixed greens spinner. Ensure your kale is dry before the subsequent stage. You can search with a paper towel and let air dry on a cooling rack until dry.

- ✓ Spot the dry kale leaves in a bowl and sprinkle on about half tablespoon avocado oil. Back rub oil into the kale leaves utilizing your fingertips.

- ✓ Sprinkle on 1 TBS dietary yeast and the entirety of your seasonings. Include another half tablespoon and rehash this procedure with well-oiled hands, kneading the dietary yeast and seasonings into the kale leaves.

- ✓ Move leaves to the preparing sheet, arrangeing in a solitary layer. Sprinkle on the remainder of the wholesome yeast and a couple of more runs of salt in the event that you wish.

✓ Prepare kale at 300°F for 7-9 mints, observing intently. All stoves are unique, so alter preparing time to the ideal surface of kale chips. Permit kale chips to cool on the search for gold mints before getting a charge out of.

CINNAMON APPLE CHIPS

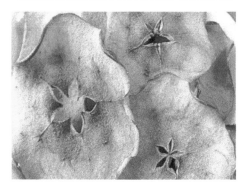

Prep Time: 5mints, Cook Time: 2hrs, Total Time: 2hrs 5mints

Servings: 4

INGREDIENTS

- ➢ 2- apples
- ➢ Cinnamon

INSTRUCTIONS

- ✓ Preheat stove to 200°F.

- ✓ Daintily cut the apples, evacuating any seeds.

- ✓ Sprinkle with cinnamon.

- ✓ Prepare for 60 mints. Flip the apples. Heat for one more hour

- ✓ Let apple chips cool, and eat!

VEGAN CARROT WAFFLES

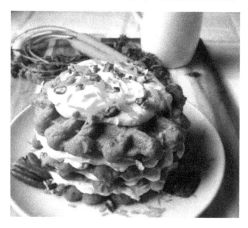

Prep Time: 10mints, Cook Time: 15mints, Total Time: 25mints

Serving: 4-6 waffles

INGREDIENTS

- 2 cups whole spelt flour or white/wheat mix
- 2 teaspoon baking powder
- 2 tablespoons ground flaxseed
- ½ teaspoon cinnamon
- 1 cup grated carrots

- 2 cups almond milk at room temperature
- ¼ cup melted coconut oil
- 1 teaspoon vanilla extract
- 2 tablespoons maple syrup
- Sea salt
- Maple syrup and/or coconut cream

✓ Preheat waffle iron.

✓ In a huge bowl, blend the flour, preparing powder, flaxseed, cinnamon, and a touch of salt.

✓ In a medium bowl, combine the ground carrots, almond milk, coconut oil, vanilla, and maple syrup. Overlay the carrot blend into the dry INGREDIENTS: and mix until simply consolidated.

✓ Scoop a suitable measure of batter onto your waffle iron and cook until the edges are marginally fresh. Present with maple syrup and the coconut cream, if utilizing.

COLD SESAME NOODLES WITH SPIRALIZED VEGETABLES

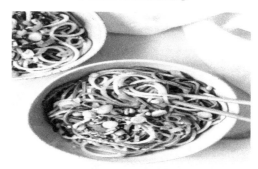

Prep Time: 20mints, Cook Time: 10mints, Total Time: 30mints

Serving: 3

INGREDIENTS

- 4- oz whole wheat spaghetti uncooked
- 1- medium-sized zucchini spiralized
- 2- large carrots spiralized
- 2- cups chickpeas
- Green onions to garnish
- Sesame seeds to garnish
- Almond Butter Sauce:
- ¼- cup almond butter
- 1- teaspoon finely grated ginger
- 1- clove garlic minced
- 2- tablespoons soy sauce
- 3- tablespoons rice vinegar

- ➤ 1- tablespoon sesame oil
- ➤ 1- tablespoon maple syrup
- ➤ 1- teaspoon lime juice
- ➤ ½- teaspoon red pepper flakes optional; omit for non-spicy version

INSTRUCTIONS

- ✓ Cook pasta as per bundle headings. Wash under virus water and put aside to cool totally.

- ✓ Part out pasta, zoodles, carrot noodles and chickpeas between four 2-cup stockpiling compartments. Sprinkle with green onions and sesame seeds.

- ✓ Mix or shake together all almond margarine sauce INGREDIENTS:, and the gap among 2 oz stockpiling holders.

- ✓ Enjoy cold. Shower with the almond adulate sauce and toss before serving.

EASY VEGAN RED LENTIL DAL

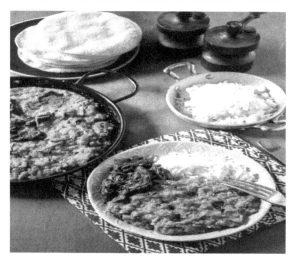

Cook Time: 15mints, Total Time: 15mints

Servings: 6

INGREDIENTS

- 3 cups of water
- 2 cups dried red lentils
- 1 15 oz can of coconut milk
- 1 tablespoon curry powder
- 2 teaspoons turmeric
- 1 teaspoon cumin
- 1 teaspoon ginger
- 1/2 teaspoon salt & pepper

INSTRUCTIONS

✓ Heat water to the point of boiling, at that factor, include lentils and coconut milk. Return mixture to a bubble at that point lessens to stew.

✓ Cook for 10 mints, till the lentils, have comfy, at that point blend in flavors and cook dinner any other 5.!

✓ Present with quinoa, cauliflower rice, white/darker rice or flatbreads!

SLOW COOKER SWEET POTATO CHICKPEA CHILI

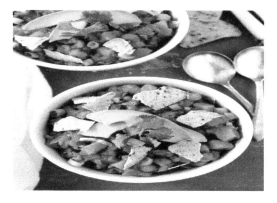

Prep Time: 30mints, Cook Time: 10hrs, Total Time: 10hrs 30mints

Servings: 8

INGREDIENTS

- Chili
- 28- oz can of diced tomatoes
- 13.5- oz can of tomato sauce 400mL
- 4- tablespoons adobo sauce
- 2- tablespoons chili powder
- 1- tsp ground cumin
- 1- tsp salt
- ½- cup stock
- 1- large sweet potato
- 4- cloves garlic
- 2- medium onions
- 2- carrots
- 19- oz of chickpeas
- After cooking:
- Juice of half a lime
- To Serve (Optional)
- Avocado
- Cilantro leaves
- Sour cream or Greek yogurt
- Tortilla chips

INSTRUCTIONS

✓ Add all INGREDIENTS: to the base of a 5-quart moderate cooker. Blend in with a spatula until totally joined.

✓ Now, the moderate cooker addition might be refrigerated medium-term, until prepared to cook.

✓ Cook in the most reduced setting for 8-10 hours.

✓ Prior to serving, delicately mix in the lime juice.

✓ Present with avocado, cilantro, yogurt/harsh cream, and tortilla chips.

VEGAN 'CHEESY' SPAGHETTI SQUASH MEAL PREP

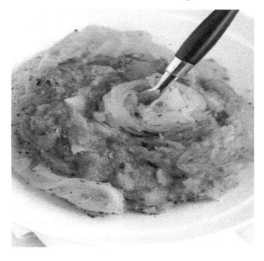

Prep Time: 15mints, Cook Time: 50mints, Total Time: 1hr 5mints

Serving: 4

INGREDIENTS

- 2 medium spaghetti squash
- 4 cups broccoli florets
- 2 tbs Coconut Oil
- 2 tbs coconut flour
- 1 cup cashews soaked in water 20 mints
- 1 cup unsweetened coconut milk
- 4 tbs nutritional yeast
- 2 tsp crushed red pepper flakes
- salt & pepper

✓ Consolidate all INGREDIENTS: with the exception of a lime squeeze in the base of a huge moderate cooker and cook low 8 for a considerable length of time.

✓ Include salt and lime, acclimate to taste.

✓ Squash everything up with a potato masher or fill in as it stands.

✓ Cooler Crockpot Meal:

✓ Join all INGREDIENTS: aside from the stock in a gallon-sized cooler sack, reusable silicone pack, or enormous supper prep holder. Evacuate however much air as could be expected.

✓ Freeze for as long as 3 months.

✓ Defrost totally, at that point add to the base of a 5-quart moderate cooker with the stock. Cook on low for 8 hours

SLOW COOKER SWEET POTATO MEXICAN QUINOA

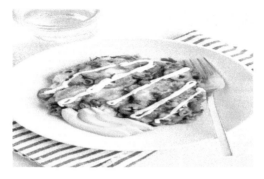

Prep Time: 10mints, Cook Time: 4hrs, Total Time: 4hrs 10mints

Serving: 6

INGREDIENTS

- 1 cup quinoa
- 1 15 oz. can black beans
- 1 15 oz. can whole kernel corn
- 1 28 oz. can crushed tomatoes
- 1 4 oz. can green chiles
- 1 large sweet potato
- 2 cups broth
- 1/2 large red onion
- 3 tablespoon chili powder
- 1 tablespoon garlic powder
- 1 tablespoon ground cumin
- 1 teaspoon paprika
- 1 tablespoon sriracha
- 2 teaspoons maple syrup
- Optional Toppings:
- fresh cilantro
- Greek yogurt
- avocado
- paprika

INSTRUCTIONS

- ✓ Find all the INGREDIENTS: in a moderate cooker and give it a decent mix.

- ✓ Spray and cook on high for around 3-4 hours or on low for 6-8.

- ✓ Sporadically mix.

MEAL PREP BALSAMIC TEMPEH & ROASTED VEGETABLE QUINOA

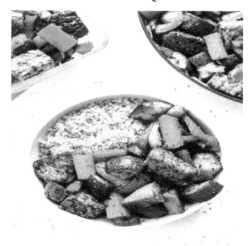

Prep Time: 5mints, Cook Time: 30mints, Total Time: 35mints

Servings: 6

INGREDIENTS

- 3- tablespoons balsamic vinegar
- 1- tablespoon olive oil
- 1- tablespoon Italian seasoning
- ½- teaspoon each of salt & pepper
- 1- package button mushrooms
- 2- medium zucchinis
- 2- carrots
- 2- red bell peppers
- 1- large shallot or red onion
- 2- packages tempeh
- 3 – 4- cups cooked quinoa

INSTRUCTIONS

- ✓ Preheat broiler to 425°F. Line a heating sheet with material and put it in a safe spot.

- ✓ Whisk together the vinegar, oil, and flavors.

- ✓ Add the vegetables and tempeh to an enormous blending bowl, at that point pour dressing over top. Toss to consolidate.

- ✓ Move everything to the heating sheet and meal for 25 - 30 mints until the vegetables are delicate and the tempeh has begun to dark-colored.

- ✓ Remove from broiler and partition equitably between holders. Include quinoa into every compartment and enable everything to cool to room temperature until ingredient and setting it in the ice chest.

VEGAN GLUTEN-FREE, DAIRY FREE

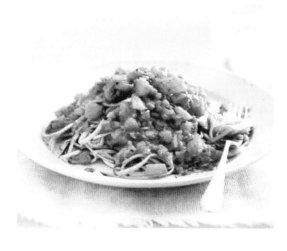

Prep Time: 5min, Cook Time: 15 min, Total Time: 20 min

Serving: 1

INGREDIENTS

- 1- wide-mouth quart mason jar with lid
- ½- cup carrot
- ½- cup julienned red pepper
- 1- teaspoon fresh ginger
- 1- teaspoon garlic
- ¼- cup green onion
- 1- cup uncooked thin rice noodles
- 1/8- cup gluten-free soy sauce
- 3- cups vegetable stock

INSTRUCTIONS

✓ In a gigantic mason, the holder incorporates carrots, red pepper, ginger, garlic, green onion, and rice noodles in a particular request.

✓ Exactly when arranged to eat, pour in soy sauce and percolating vegetable stock.

✓ Another other option: When arranged to eat pour in soy sauce, concentrated liquid vegetable stock and 3 cups of gurgling high temp water.

✓ Fix top onto the compartment and grant to sit for 10-15 mints, or until veggies and noodles are sensitive.

LEMON COCONUT CHIA MUFFINS

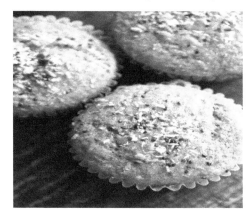

Prep Time: 1hr, Cook Time: 30mints, Total Time: hr 30mints

Serving: 10

INGREDIENTS

- ➢ Wet:
- ➢ 1- cup full-fat coconut milk
- ➢ zest of a lemon
- ➢ juice of 2 lemons
- ➢ 2 to 3 tbsp chia seeds
- ➢ ½ to 2/3 cup sugar raw, cane or other
- ➢ ¼- tsp or more turmeric
- ➢ ½- tsp vanilla extract optional

- ➢ Dry:
- ➢ 1- cup whole wheat flour
- ➢ ¼- cup unbleached white flour
- ➢ 2 to 3 tbsp dried coconut flakes
- ➢ ½- tsp baking soda
- ➢ ¾- tsp baking powder
- ➢ ¼- tsp salt

INSTRUCTIONS

- ✓ Blend all the wet INGREDIENTS: until sugar is very much consolidated. Refrigerate for in any event an hour to hydrate the chia seeds.

- ✓ Line a biscuit skillet with biscuit liners.Preheat the stove to 350 degrees F.

- ✓ In a bowl, whisk all the dry INGREDIENTS:. Add to the wet and blend to join. The hitter ought to be to some degree flowy however not runny. In the event that excessively runny, include a couple of tbsp more flours and blend in.

- ✓ Include more turmeric if necessary. Overlap in dried organic product or nuts, candy-coated lemon or blueberries now.

- ✓ Drop the hitter into a lined biscuit skillet. Sprinkle coconut and chia seeds on top. Prepare at 350 degrees F/170°c for 26 to 28 mints.

- ✓ Cool for 5 mints in the container then a couple of moments on the counter before serving. The biscuits can be kept on the counter for as long as 2 days

EASY VEGAN WAFFLES

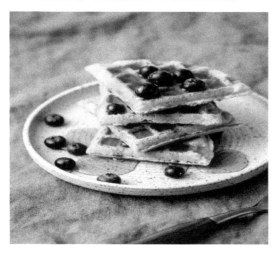

Prep Time: 5mints, Cook Time: 10mints, Total Time: 15mints

Serving: 4 waffles

INGREDIENTS

- 1 ½- cups spelled flour
- 2- heaping tablespoons coconut
- 2- teaspoons baking powder
- 1 ½- cups unsweetened vanilla almond milk
- 3- tablespoons grape seed
- pinch of mineral salt

INSTRUCTIONS

- ✓ Preheat waffle creator as indicated by producers' INGREDIENTS:. Additionally, preheat stove to 200 degrees F., for keeping the waffles warm.

- ✓ In a medium-sized blending bowl, consolidate the flour, sugar, heating powder, oil, and non-dairy milk, blend well, until the greater part of the flour bumps is no more.

- ✓ On the off chance that utilizing this Cuisinart waffle creator or one comparable, utilizing a 1/2 estimating cup, gather up the batter and pour in the focal point of the warmed waffle producer plate. Close the spread and hold up until the light turns green.

- ✓ Tenderly evacuate and spot on a wire rack in the broiler until the rest of the waffles are made.

- ✓ Serve your waffles with crisp blueberries, strawberries, raspberries or blackberries, top with unadulterated maple syrup, or this simple custom made Blueberry Compote.

- ✓ Store extra waffles in the fridge for as long as seven days, or store in the cooler for up to 1-2 months. At the point when prepared to eat, pop them in the toaster stove.

SIMPLE VEGAN AVOCADO TOAST RECIPE

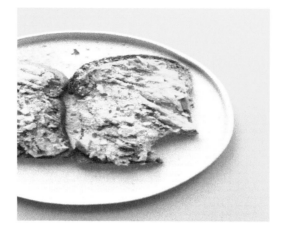

Prep Time: 5mints, Cook Time:10mints, Total Time: 15mints

Servings: 2

INGREDIENTS

- 4- slices multi-grain bread
- 1- ripe avocado
- A handful of pea shoots salad
- ½- lime
- A pinch of salt
- A pinch of pepper
- 1 ½- cups cooked chickpeas
- 2- tablespoons olive oil
- 6- sun-dried tomatoes in olive oil
- 1- teaspoon smoked paprika
- A pinch of salt

INSTRUCTIONS

- ✓ Make a glue with the sun-dried tomatoes by hacking them as finely as could be allowed.

- ✓ Following 5 mints, sprinkle the chickpeas with the smoked paprika and a spot of salt to taste.

- ✓ Mix well and include the sun-got tomato glue and turn dry the warmth.

- ✓ Toast the bread until brilliant and fresh.

- ✓ Cut the avocado into equal parts, crush it with a fork. Sprinkle with the lime juice and a spot of salt and pepper.

- ✓ Top with the warm chickpeas and pea shoots serving of mixed greens. Enjoy

HOMEMADE OVEN BAKED BEANS

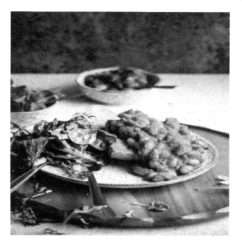

Prep Time: 10mints, Cook Time: 1hr 30mints, Total Time: 1hr 40mints

Servings: 4

INGREDIENTS

- 2 Red Onions
- 3 Cloves of Garlic
- 1 Red Chilli
- 1 tbsp olive oil
- 1 tsp Smoked Paprika
- 1 tsp Chilli Flakes
- 1/2 tsp Ground Cumin
- 1 jar Tomato Passata
- 14- oz Pinto Beans
- 2 tbsp Balsamic Vinegar
- 1 tsp Molasses
- 4-5 sprigs Fresh Thyme

INSTRUCTIONS

- ✓ Preheat the stove to 170°C.

- ✓ Shakers the onion, and finely hack the stew and garlic. Spot into an enormous, stove verification cooking plate, blend in with the olive oil and flavors, spread with foil and dish for 20 mints.

- ✓ Following 20 mints, remove from the stove, include the remainder of the INGREDIENTS: to the cooking plate and mix completely.

- ✓ Broil for an additional 45 mints, revealed this time, at that point remove from the broiler and mix. If necessary, mean 1/4 cup of water to disperse the sauce.

QUINOA SALAD WITH AVOCADO, BEANS, CORN PEACHES

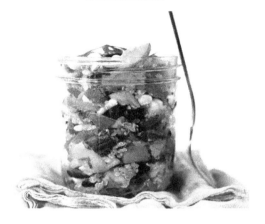

Prep Time: 10mints, Total Time: 10mints

Serving: 2

INGREDIENTS

- ¼- cup extra virgin olive oil
- ¼- cup fresh lime juice
- 1- clove garlic
- 2- cups cooked quinoa
- 15- oz. black beans
- 15- oz. kidney beans
- ½- red onion
- 1- red bell pepper
- 1- Persian cucumber
- 2- ears corn
- ¼- cup fresh cilantro
- 2- peaches
- 1-2 avocados

INSTRUCTIONS

✓ In a bit bowl or container, whisk together the olive oil, lime juice, and garlic.

✓ In a large serving bowl, mix together the quinoa, beans, onion, ringer pepper, cucumber, corn, and cilantro

✓ Sprinkle with the dressing and blend to cover.

✓ Include the peaches and avocados and either blend in or orchestrate on the pinnacle.

✓ Sprinkle a touch lime squeezed over the peaches and avocados to keep new if leaving on top.

✓ Spread with grasp wrap and refrigerate until organized to eat.

MAKE-AHEAD SUPER GREEN VEGAN QUINOA BURRITOS

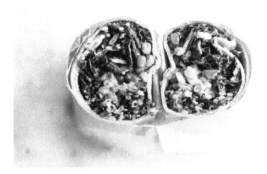

Prep Time: 10mints, Cooking Time: 25mints, Total Time: 35mints

Serving: 3

INGREDIENTS

- 1 avocado
- 2 cloves garlic
- 4 scallion
- a handful of chives, basil, and/or cilantro
- 1/4 cup tahini or almond butter
- 1/4 cup water
- tablespoons lemon juice
- salt or coconut aminos
- 1 serrano chile pepper
- 2 bunches of kale
- 6 multi-grain or spinach tortillas
- 3 cups cooked mung beans
- 3 cups cooked quinoa
- optional: toasted pepitas, hemp seeds

- ✓ Consolidate the avocado, garlic, scallion, herbs, tahini, water, lemon juice, salt, and serrano in a blender or nourishment processor and heartbeat till wealthy. Move to a container.

- ✓ Spot the kale in an significant bowl, and include around half of the dressing to it. Back rub with your arms until the kale is pleasantly covered and beginning to fall apiece.

- ✓ Spot one tortilla on the counter and load up with around half cup of the quinoa, half of cup of the mung beans, some liberal dabs of the dressing, a bunch of the kale combo, and a sprinkling of pepitas and hemp seeds. Crease and roll, and in a while rehash with the last burritos.

- ✓ Enclose every via cloth paper, and later on foil if you're looking ahead to ingesting later. You can freeze in products, enveloped through cloth, and afterward foil in massive plastic packs.

MINTS CHOCOLATE CHIP

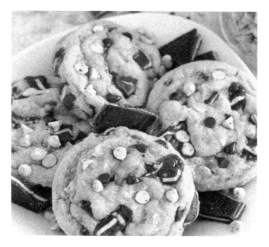

Prep Time: 10mints, Total time: 25mints

Serving: 2

INGREDIENTS

- ➢ 1- medium banana
- ➢ ½- of an avocado
- ➢ 2- tablespoons cacao nibs
- ➢ 2- tablespoons cacao powder
- ➢ ¼- cup fresh mints
- ➢ 1- cup spinach
- ➢ 1 ½- cups Almond Breeze Unsweetened Chocolate Almondmilk

✓ Include the banana, avocado, cacao nibs, cacao powder, mints and spinach into a little pack and spot in the cooler.

✓ At the point when prepared to mix, include the smoothie pack, alongside the almond milk, and mix until smooth.

VEGAN WALNUT DRIED APRICOT BARS

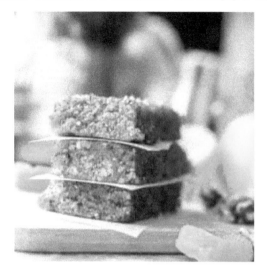

Prep Time: 15mints, Total Time: 15mints

Serving: 6

INGREDIENTS

- 1- cup walnuts
- ½- cup dried apricot
- ¼- cup goji berries
- 1- tablespoon lemon juice
- 4- dates pits removed and

  softened in water for 10 mints
- 1- lemon zested
- 1- tablespoon chia seeds
- 1- tablespoon hemp seeds

INSTRUCTIONS

✓ Absorb dates warm water for 10 mints to loosen up then a chunk. Channel the water.

✓ Consolidate all INGREDIENTS: in nourishment processor and manner till almost clean

✓ Pat bars right into a heating plate and freezes for 10-15 mints.

✓ Cut into bars and keep within the fridge.

CHOCOLATE PEANUT BUTTER PROTEIN BAKED OATMEAL CUPS

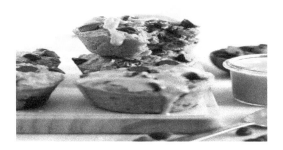

Prep Time: 10mints, Cook Time: 25mints, Total Time: 35mints

Serving: 4

INGREDIENTS

- 2- tbsp chia seeds + 6 tbsp water
- 3- medium to large ripe bananas
- 1- cup Silk unsweetened cashew milk
- ¼- cup creamy peanut butter
- ¼- cup pure maple syrup
- ½- tsp vanilla extract
- 1- scoop chocolate plant-based protein powder
- 3- cups old fashioned oats
- 2- tbsp cocoa powder
- 1- tbsp baking powder
- pinch salt

INSTRUCTIONS

✓ Preheat broiler to 350F. Shower biscuit tin with cooking splash.

✓ In a little bowl, mix collectively chia seeds and water to make "chia eggs." Alternatively, you could utilize 2 sizable eggs. Put in a secure spot.

✓ Spot bananas in a big bowl and pound with a fork. Include cashew milk, nutty unfold, discretionary maple syrup or stevia, and vanilla and mix until very lots combined. Mix in chia eggs.

✓ Include protein powder, oats, cocoa powder, getting ready powder, and salt. Mix till consolidated.

✓ Spoon blend similarly into the biscuit tin. You can fill the tins to the pinnacle. You may additionally have some closing hitter. Prepare for 25 mints.

✓ Remove from range and cool in a container on a wire rack. When totally cool, shop in an impenetrable compartment within the cooler

VEGAN NO-BAKE PUMPKIN CHEESECAKE BITES RECIPE

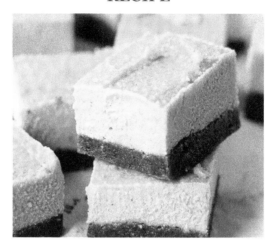

Prep Time: 1hr 5mints, Cooking Time: 2hrs 10mints, Total Time: 3hrs 15mints

Serving: 16-20 squares

INGREDIENTS

- Crust:
- 1 cup Pitted Dates
- 1/2 cup Almond Flour
- 1 tbsp Organic Cacao Powder
- 2 tsp vanilla extract
- 1 tbsp almond milk

- Cheesecake layer:
- 1 1/2 cups Raw Cashews
- 1/3 cup maple syrup
- 1/3 cup canned pumpkin
- 1 tsp Pumpkin Spice Blend

✓ Absorb the cashews water for 60 mints. Dispose of the water. Line a portion of heating dish with material paper and put it in a safe spot.

✓ Spot the covering INGREDIENTS: in your blender and heartbeat until the blend meets up; this should take around 1 moment. Press this blend uniformly onto the base of the readied portion heating container and spot it in the cooler while you set up the cheesecake besting.

✓ Spot the cheesecake INGREDIENTS: in your nourishment processor and heartbeat until smooth.

✓ Pour the cheesecake blend over the outside layer in the preparing skillet and spread it equally. Freeze the sweet for at any rate 2 hours.

✓ Cut the cheesecake into squares before serving. Keep scraps shrouded in the cooler for as long as 3 months.

5 MINUTE PROTEIN PEANUT BUTTER ENERGY BITES

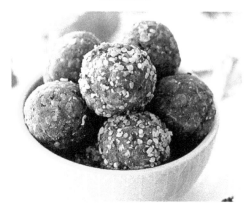

Prep Time: 5mints, Total Time: 5mints

Serving: 10

INGREDIENTS

- 1/2 cup natural drippy peanut butter
- 1/4 cup honey
- 1 teaspoon vanilla extract
- 1/3 cup protein powder of choice
- 1/3 cup flaxseed meal
- 1/2 cup rolled oats
- 1/2 teaspoon cinnamon
- 1 tablespoon chia seeds
- 1 tablespoon mini chocolate chips
- Optional
- 1/4 cup unsweetened shredded coconut

INSTRUCTIONS

✓ In the bowl of a nourishment processor, encompass the nutty spread, nectar, vanilla, protein powder, flaxseed meal, oats, cinnamon and chia seeds.

✓ Heartbeat collectively till very a good deal joined. Include chocolate chips and heartbeat a couple of extra events.

✓ Utilize a medium treat scoop or your fingers to get aggregate and fold into 10 balls, region in a water/air proof holder.

✓ To make without a nourishment processor: add moist INGREDIENTS: to a medium bowl, the mixture to consolidate.

✓ Include dry INGREDIENTS: and integrate them still joined.

✓ Since all nutty unfold/nut margarine textures are specific and relying upon what protein powder you use

✓ You can want to include greater nut margarine or sugar to allow the balls to live together.

MANGO-DATE ENERGY BITES

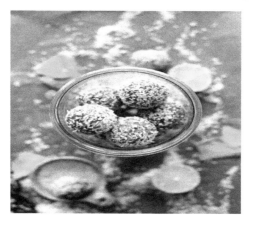

Prep Time: 5mints, Total Time: 15mints

Servings: 20

INGREDIENTS

- ➢ 2- cups pitted whole dates
- ➢ 1- cup raw cashews
- ➢ 1- cup dried mango
- ➢ ¼- teaspoon salt

INSTRUCTIONS

- ✓ Procedure dates, cashews, mango and salt in a nourishment processor until finely hacked.

- ✓ Structure into around 20 balls, utilizing 2 tablespoons each

DINNER

ASPARAGUS & MUSHROOM VEGAN QUICHE

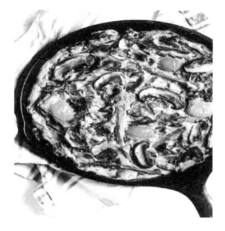

Prep Time: 10mints, Cook Time: 40mints, Total Time: 50mints

Serving: 4

INGREDIENTS

- 2 cups asparagus
- 8 ounces mushrooms
- 1 cup tomatoes
- 2 cups kale or spinach
- 1 12.3-ounce package silken tofu
- 1 cup chickpea flour
- 1/4 cup nutritional yeast
- 2 tablespoons soy sauce
- 1 teaspoon ground thyme
- 1 teaspoon ground oregano
- 1/2 teaspoon ground turmeric
- 1/2 teaspoon Kala namak
- 1/4 teaspoon black pepper

INSTRUCTIONS

- ✓ Preheat stove to 350F. Delicately oil a medium cast-iron skillet.

- ✓ In a wok or huge skillet, warm a little water or oil over medium warmth. Include asparagus; cook for 4-5 mints. Include mushrooms, tomatoes, and kale; cook for 5 additional mints, until vegetables are delicate.

- ✓ In a nourishment processor or blender, include tofu, chickpea flour, healthful yeast, soy sauce, thyme, oregano, turmeric, salt, and pepper. Mix until smooth.

- ✓ Remove vegetables from heat; pour in the tofu blend and mix to join. Empty the blend into the skillet.

- ✓ Prepare for 40 mints. Remove; put in a safe spot for 10 mints before serving.

VEGAN AFRICAN PEANUT STEW

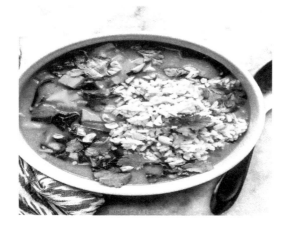

Prep Time: 15mints, Cook Time: 6hrs, Total Time: 6 hrs 15mints

Serving: 4

INGREDIENTS

- 15- oz can of chickpeas
- 4- cups vegetable stock
- ½- teaspoon salt
- 1- teaspoon cumin
- ½- teaspoon ground coriander
- ¼- teaspoon cayenne
- 15- oz can of diced tomatoes
- 4-5- cups sweet potatoes
- ½- cup all-natural peanut butter
- 1- onion
- 4- cloves garlic
- 1- inch ginger
- Just before serving
- 4- handfuls spinach

✓ Join all INGREDIENTS: in a 6-quart moderate cooker and cook on low for 6-8 hours.

✓ Blend in the spinach and cook for 15 mints.

✓ Squash the sweet potato until the stew is thickened. Enjoy!

✓ To hoard ahead and freeze:

✓ Get all INGREDIENTS: together except for the stock and spinach in an enormous cooler pack. Press out anyway a lot of air as could be normal and freeze level. Freeze for up to 3 months.

✓ Defrost absolutely and cook as demonstrated by the headings above.

VEGAN PORTOBELLO FAJITA MEAL PREP BOWLS

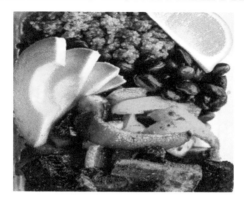

Prep Time: 20mints, Cook Time: 20mints, Total Time: 40mints

Serving: 5

INGREDIENTS

- Spice Blend
- 1 teaspoon onion powder
- 1 teaspoon garlic powder
- 1 teaspoon chili powder
- 1 teaspoon ground cumin
- 1 teaspoon salt
- 1 teaspoon red pepper flakes
- 3/4 cup quinoa uncooked
- 2 tablespoons olive oil
- 4 portobello mushrooms cut into strips
- 2 bell peppers
- 1 zucchini
- 1/2 red onion
- After cooking:
- 1 cup black beans
- lime wedges

✓ Warmth broiler to 425°F.

✓ Mix together the zest mix.

✓ Include half of the zest mix to the cooking fluid with the quinoa, at that point cook quinoa as indicated by bundle bearings. Permit cooling.

✓ Toss the vegetables in olive oil and sprinkle with the rest of the zest mix. Arrange on a couple of preparing sheets.

✓ Heat veggies for 15 mints, give them a mix and come back to the stove in the event that they are not cooked exactly as you would prefer. I cooked for 20 mints in all-out time. Cool.

✓ The gap into four supper prep compartments: quinoa, veggies, dark beans, and extra INGREDIENTS: like salsa or yogurt whenever wanted. We adored our own presented with crisply cut avocado

VEGAN GINGER TERIYAKI STIR FRY

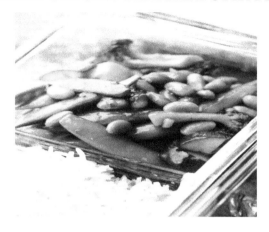

Prep Time: 15mints, Cook Time: 15mints, Total Time: 30mints

Servings: 4

INGREDIENTS

- 1 tablespoon olive oil
- 4 cups vegetables broccoli
- 2 cups edamame shelled
- 1 tablespoon ginger
- 1 clove garlic
- Vegan Teriyaki Sauce
- 3 tablespoons reduced-sodium soy sauce
- 5 tablespoons maple syrup
- 1 teaspoon sesame oil
- 2 teaspoons corn starch
- 1/2 teaspoon red pepper flakes
- 1 teaspoon sake

- ✓ Shake together all-veggie lover teriyaki sauce INGREDIENTS: and put in a safe spot.

- ✓ Warmth oil over medium warmth in a massive skillet.

- ✓ Include the vegetables and edamame. Cook for 5-7 mints, blending sporadically till mellowed.

- ✓ Give the veggie lover teriyaki sauce a respectable shake, at that factor empty it into the skillet. Cook for 1-2 mints till sauce is thickened and all veggies are included.

- ✓ Serve promptly over rice.

MAKE-AHEAD CHICKPEA BUTTERNUT SQUASH FAJITAS

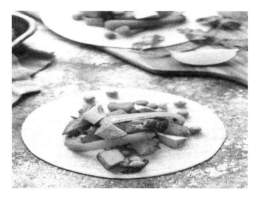

Prep Time: 20mints, Cook Time: 25mints, Total Time: 45mints

Servings: 4 -6

INGREDIENTS

- 4 cups butternut squash
- 1 19 oz can chickpeas
- 1 red onion
- 2 bell peppers
- 1 tablespoon maple syrup
- 1/2 teaspoon salt
- 1 tablespoon chili powder
- 1.5 teaspoon cumin
- 1.5 teaspoon paprika
- 1/2 teaspoon garlic powder
- 2 tablespoons olive oil
- juice from 1 lime
- To Serve:
- 8-12 six-inch tortillas
- Greek yogurt
- Avocado
- Cilantro
- Salsa

✓ Consolidate all INGREDIENTS: in an uncompromising cooler sack.

✓ Shake until everything is equally consolidated.

✓ Freeze for as long as a multi month.

✓ To Bake: Thaw totally before preparing.

✓ Warmth stove to 425°F. Spread all fajita INGREDIENTS: out uniformly on a huge preparing dish.

✓ Prepare for 25 mints, flipping everything part of the way through.

GRILLED VEGGIE & BLACK BEAN MEAL PREP BOWLS

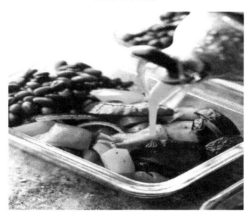

Prep Time: 15mints, Cook Time: 30mints, Total Time: 45mints

Servings: 4

INGREDIENTS

- BBQ Vinaigrette
- 2 tablespoons white wine vinegar
- 3 tablespoons bbq sauce
- 2 teaspoons honey
- 1 teaspoon lime
- 1/4 teaspoon chili powder
- 1/4 tsp salt

- Meal Prep Bowls:
- 3/4 cup uncooked quinoa
- 1 tablespoon olive oil
- salt & pepper
- 1 medium zucchini
- 2 bell peppers
- 1/2 red onion
- 19 oz can of black beans

INSTRUCTIONS

- ✓ Shake together regardless of vinaigrette INGREDIENTS: and set.

- ✓ Cook quinoa as per bundle headings and permit to cool.

- ✓ Warmth grill over medium-high warmth.

- ✓ Toss the veggies with olive oil and salt and pepper in a huge bowl. Arrange on a vegetable barbecuing container and flame broil for 10-15 mints, flipping like clockwork.

- ✓ Separation into every one of four 2 cup stockpiling holders the quinoa, barbecued veggies, and dark beans.

- ✓ Shower with vinaigrette.

- ✓ Store in the cooler for as long as 4 days, and serve cold

SLOW COOKER CHICKPEA TORTILLA SOUP

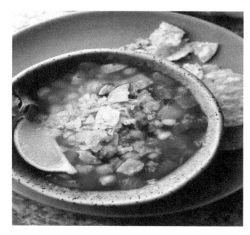

Prep Time: 10mints, Cook Time: 4hrs, Total Time: 4hrs 10mints

Servings: 4 -6

INGREDIENTS

- 1 cup of salsa
- 1 teaspoon cumin
- 1 teaspoon chili powder
- 1/4 teaspoon salt
- 1 19 oz can of chickpeas
- 1 15 oz can of corn
- 1 onion chopped
- 3 cloves garlic
- 4 cups vegetable or chicken stock
- Before Serving:
- 1 tablespoon lime juice
- Toppings:
- tortilla chips
- avocado
- greek yogurt
- cilantro leaves

- ✓ Shake together regardless of vinaigrette INGREDIENTS: and set.

- ✓ Cook quinoa as per bundle bearings and permit to cool.

- ✓ Warmth grill over medium-high warmth.

- ✓ Toss the veggies with olive oil and salt and pepper in an enormous bowl. Organize on a vegetable flame broiling dish and barbecue for 10-15 mints, flipping like clockwork.

- ✓ Partition into every one of four 2 cup stockpiling holders the quinoa, flame-broiled veggies, and dark beans.

- ✓ Shower with vinaigrette.

- ✓ Store in the cooler for as long as 4 days, and serve cold

SLOW COOKER BUTTERNUT SQUASH LENTIL CURRY

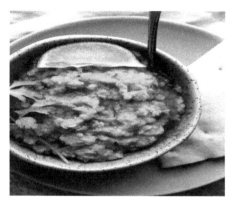

Prep Time: 20mints, Cook Time: 8hrs, Total Time: 8hrs 20mints

Servings: 8

INGREDIENTS

- 2 cups red lentils
- 4 cups butternut squash
- 1 onion
- 2 cloves garlic
- 2 tablespoons fresh ginger
- 1 tablespoon curry powder
- 2 teaspoons ground coriander
- 2 teaspoons garam masala
- 2 teaspoons turmeric
- 2 teaspoons ground cumin
- 1 teaspoon salt
- 13.5 oz coconut milk
- 19 oz diced tomatoes
- 3 cups stock
- After cooking:
- 1/2 lime
- salt

- ✓ Consolidate all INGREDIENTS: apart from lime squeeze within the base of an extensive slight cooker and cook low eight for pretty a long time.

- ✓ Include salt and lime, alternate in accordance with flavor.

- ✓ Squash everything up with a potato masher or fill in its gift situation.

- ✓ Cooler Crockpot Meal:

- ✓ Consolidate all INGREDIENTS: except the stock in a gallon-sized cooler percent, reusable silicone sack, or great meal prep compartment. Remove however tons air as may be anticipated.

- ✓ Freeze for as long as three months.

- ✓ Defrost totally, at that point add to the bottom of a five-quart moderate cooker with the inventory. Cook on low for 8 hours

TOFU BURRITO BOWL MEAL PREP

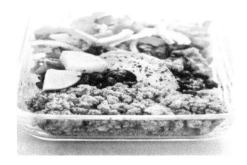

Prep Time: 5mints, Cook Time: 10mints, Total Time: 15mints

Serving: 5

INGREDIENTS

- 14 oz. extra firm tofu
- 2 Tablespoons olive oil
- 1/2 teaspoon sea salt
- 1/2 teaspoon pepper
- 1/2 teaspoon chipotle powder
- 1/2 teaspoon chili powder
- 1/2 teaspoon paprika
- 1/4 teaspoon garlic powder
- 1/8 teaspoon cayenne
- Toppings:
- Greens – romaine, spinach, kale, etc.
- Avocado or guacamole
- Black beans or refried beans
- Red onion
- Tomatoes or salsa
- Cilantro

INSTRUCTIONS

- ✓ Channel tofu. Evacuate however a whole lot abundance fluid as may be expected by using squeezing between paper towels.

- ✓ In a good-sized skillet, heat oil to medium and consist of the rectangular of tofu. Utilize a spoon or spatula to "curb" the tofu. Include seasonings and hold "hacking" and mixing until the entirety of the tofu is ready.

- ✓ Cook eight-10 mints, till tofu is warmed throughout.

- ✓ Part tofu into supper prep compartments and encompass desired INGREDIENTS:.

- ✓ Store in the refrigerator for so long as 10 days

HEALTHY THAI COCONUT QUINOA BOWLS

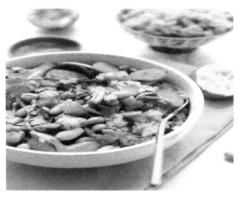

Prep Time: 15mints, Cook Time: 30mints, Total Time: 45mints

Serving: 4

INGREDIENTS

- For the Coconut Quinoa:
- Roasted Veggies
- 1 large sweet potato
- 2 cups carrots
- 1 tablespoon minced garlic
- 2 tablespoons EVOO
- salt and pepper
- Purple Cabbage Slaw
- 1 cup purple cabbage
- 1 cup edamame
- 1 small red pepper

- 1 tablespoon low-sodium tamari
- 2 tablespoons EVOO
- 1 lime
- 1 tablespoon maple syrup
- 1/4 teaspoon garlic powder
- 1/4 teaspoon ginger powder
- 1/4 teaspoon dried orange peel
- Toppings:

- ➢ peanut butter
- ➢ peanuts
- ➢ fresh cilantro

- ✓ Spot diced vegetables on a making ready sheet and shower with EVOO. At that point, encompass minced garlic and season with salt and pepper. Toss. Cook at 400°F for 25-30 mints or until you can penetrate the veggies with a fork.

- ✓ For the Purple Cabbage Slaw:

- ✓ Spot crimson cabbage, edamame, and pink pepper in a bowl. Put in a safe spot. Make your dressing by using whisking collectively EVOO, lime juice, soy sauce, maple syrup, ginger, garlic, and dried orange strip. At that point, toss veggies in dressing.

SOUTHWEST SWEET POTATO VEGAN MEAL PREP BOWLS

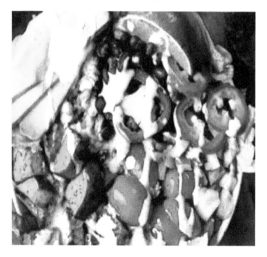

Prep Time: 15mints, Cook Time: 25mints, Total Time: 40mints

Servings: 4

- 1- large sweet potato
- 3-4- tablespoons olive oil
- 1- teaspoon southwest seasoning
- Garlic powder
- Salt & pepper

- 12- fluid ounce sweet corn drained
- 19- fluid ounce black beans
- Juice of ½- lime + wedges for serving
- ½- teaspoon ground cumin

INSTRUCTIONS

✓ Preheat broiler to 400F and move the rack to the top third of the stove.

✓ Prep your sweet potato and add the slice up pieces to a foil-lined heating sheet. Sprinkle the pieces with the southwest flavoring, garlic powder, and salt and pepper, and toss with 2-3 tablespoons of olive oil. You need each piece covered in oil yet not dribbling with it. Prepare for 25 mints or until delicate.

✓ In the meantime, including the corn, beans, lime juice, 1 tablespoon of olive oil, cumin, and salt and pepper to a little bowl. Toss.

✓ When your sweet potatoes are done, similarly isolate them and the corn/bean blend between the four Tupperware holders. Add a wedge of lime to every holder. I recommend eating the dinner prep bowls inside 5 days.

10-MINUTE CHICKPEA CURRY

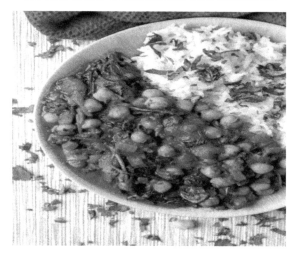

Prep Time: 2mints, Cook Time: 8mints, Total Time: 10mints

Servings: 4

INGREDIENTS

- 2 cans chickpeas
- 1 can coconut milk
- 2 teaspoon garam masala
- 2 teaspoon turmeric
- 1 teaspoon ginger powder
- 1/2 teaspoon chili flakes
- 1 medium-size onion
- 2 cloves of garlic
- 1 tablespoon olive oil
- 10 oz fresh baby spinach
- salt
- 4 lemon wedges
- Fresh coriander

INSTRUCTIONS

- ✓ Warmth the oil in an enormous dish. At the point when the oil smoking hot lower the warmth and include the flavors

- ✓ Following a couple of moments include the hacked onions and the minced garlic.

- ✓ When the onion and garlic are brilliant tans include the chickpeas and the coconut milk. Add salt to taste.

- ✓ Cook for 5 mints at that point include the washed crisp spinach, mix well and spread.

- ✓ Let the spinach shrink for a few mints. What's more, it's prepared to serve.

- ✓ You can include a sprinkle of crisp lemon juice and some new slashed coriander in the event that you like. Be that as it may, it's not fundamental.

- ✓ This curry is delectable with basmati rice or naan bread.

EASY VEGAN RED LENTIL DAL

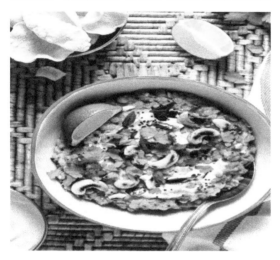

Cook Time: 15mints, Total Time: 15mints

Servings: 6

INGREDIENTS

- 3- cups of water
- 2- cups dried red lentils
- 15- oz of coconut milk
- 1- tablespoon curry powder
- 2- teaspoons turmeric
- 1- teaspoon cumin
- 1- teaspoon ginger
- ½- teaspoon salt & pepper

INSTRUCTIONS

- ✓ Heat water to the point of boiling, at that factor, include lentils and coconut milk. Return mixture to a bubble at that point decreases to stew.

- ✓ Cook for 10 mints, till the lentils, have mollified, at that factor blend in flavors and cook dinner any other five.

- ✓ Present with quinoa, cauliflower rice, white/dark colored rice or flatbreads!

MEAL PREP SESAME TOFU QUINOA BOWLS

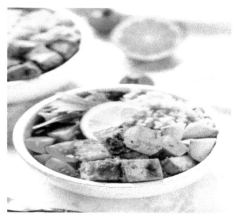

Prep Time: 10mints, Cook Time: 30mints, Total Time: 40mints

Servings: 4

INGREDIENTS

- 1- lb green beans
- 1- block extra firm tofu
- 4-cups broccoli crowns
- 2- cups cooked quinoa
- For the dressing:
- ¼- cup toasted sesame oil
- 2- tablespoons gluten-free tamari
- 1- teaspoon tapioca starch
- ½- teaspoon Organic garlic powder
- ½- teaspoon Organic ginger
- ¼ - ½- teaspoon Organic crushed pepper flakes

INSTRUCTIONS

✓ Preheat the stove to 375°F.

✓ Cut the green beans down the middle and arrange them
   alongside 33% of a heating sheet. Cut the tofu into
   scaled-down pieces and put it on the preparing sheet
   also. At long last, arrange the broccoli alongside the last
   third of the heating sheet.

✓ Whisk together the dressing INGREDIENTS: until
   cover and pour up the veggies and tofu. Mix together
   until everything is covered. Prepare on the inside track
   for 25 - 30 mints, until the veggies are pleasant and
   broiled.

✓ Gather your dishes: include 1/2 cup of quinoa to each,
   alongside 1/4 of the veggies and tofu. Shower with extra
   tamari and hot sauce whenever wanted!

MEDITERRANEAN VEGAN MEAL PREP BOWLS

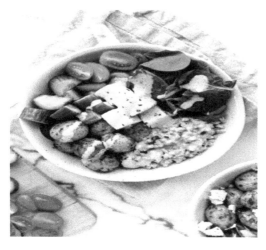

Prep Time: 10mints, Total Time: 30mints

Servings: 4 bowls

INGREDIENTS

- ¾- cup uncooked quinoa
- 19- fluid ounce chickpeas
- 2- Persian cucumbers
- Handful little tomatoes
- 2- tablespoons red onions
- Kalamata olives
- Hummus
- Optional:
- Olive oil
- Lemon juice

INSTRUCTIONS

✓ Cook quinoa as indicated by bundle headings.

✓ In the meantime, prep your different INGREDIENTS: and partition them similarly between the 4 dishes.

✓ Once the quinoa has cooled, add it to each bowl.

✓ Discretionary: sprinkle a touch of olive oil and crush some lemon squeezed over each bowl.

MEAL-PREP QUINOA BURRITO BOWLS

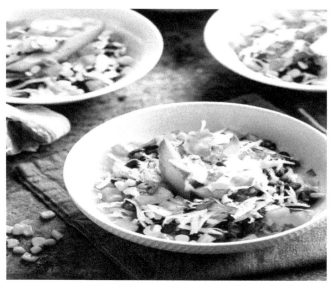

Prep Time: 15mints, Total Time: 15mints

Servings: 5

INGREDIENTS

- 3 cups cooked quinoa
- 1 15 oz can black beans
- 1 cup corn fresh or frozen
- 1/2 cup chopped cilantro
- 1 teaspoon cumin
- 1/2 teaspoon salt
- Juice of 1 lime
- 2 heads of romaine
- 1/2 cup salsa
- 3 avocados halved
- Lime slivers optional

INSTRUCTIONS

- ✓ Set up the quinoa serving of blended vegetables with the aid of consolidating the quinoa, beans, corn, cilantro, flavors and lime squeeze in a widespread bowl. Mix together until joined.

- ✓ Utilizing 5 glass compartments, include cups of romaine, half cups of quinoa mixture, 1 - 2 tablespoons of salsa and half of an avocado.

- ✓ Embellishment with lime wedges and a sprinkle extra cilantro every time desired. Seal booths and noticed inside the ice chest for so long as five days.

SUPER SIMPLE VEGAN BURRITO BOWL

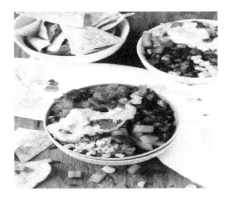

Prep Time: 5mints, Cook Time: 15mints, Total Time: 20mints

Serving: 4

INGREDIENTS

- For the Burrito Bowl:
- 1 15 oz can black beans
- 8 oz frozen corn kernels
- 2 cups dry instant brown rice
- 12 oz jar Salsa
- 1 red bell pepper
- Handful cilantro

- Creamy Avocado Dressing:
- 1 ripe avocado
- 1/3 cup vegan sour cream
- 1 tbsp lime juice
- 1 tsp cumin
- 1/2 tsp chili powder
- salt and pepper
- 2-3 tbsp nondairy milk to thin

- ✓ For the Creamy Avocado Dressing:

- ✓ Consolidate all INGREDIENTS:, other than the nondairy milk, in a touch bowl and blend properly to sign up for. Include 1 tbsp nondairy milk immediately and blend until you arrive at your ideal consistency.

- ✓ For the Burrito Bowls:

- ✓ Cook the instant rice as in keeping with package headings. At the point whilst the rice is finished, add to a similar pot the darkish beans, corn, and salsa.

- ✓ Cook over medium warmth, mixing periodically till warmed through, around five mints.

- ✓ Take off warmth, consist of ringer peppers and cilantro if making use of. Pour in Creamy Avocado Dressing and be a part of it.

- ✓ Present with tortilla chips or over hacked Romaine lettuce.

SOUTHWEST SWEET POTATO VEGAN MEAL PREP BOWLS

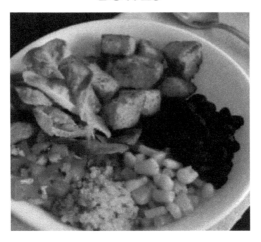

Prep Time: 15mints, Cook Time: 25mints, Total Time: 40mints

Servings: 4

- 1-enormous sweet potato
- 3-4-tablespoons olive oil
- 1-teaspoon southwest flavoring
- Garlic powder

- Salt and pepper
- 12-ounce sweet corn
- 19-ounce dark beans
- 1/2 lime Juice
- ½-teaspoon ground cumin

- ✓ Preheat oven to 400F and pass the rack to the top third of the oven.

- ✓ Prep your sweet potato and add the reduce-up pieces to a foil-coated baking sheet. Sprinkle the pieces with the southwest seasoning, garlic powder, and salt & pepper, and toss with 2-3 tablespoons of olive oil. You want each piece lined in oil however no longer dripping with it. Bake for 25 mints or until soft.

- ✓ Meanwhile, add the corn, beans, lime juice, 1 tablespoon of olive oil, cumin, and salt & pepper to a small bowl. Toss.

- ✓ Once your sweet potatoes are completed, similarly divide them and the corn/bean mixture among the four Tupperware boxes. Add a wedge of lime to every container. I advocate ingesting the meal prep bowls within 5 days.

HERBED CHEESE STUFFED MINI SWEET PEPPERS

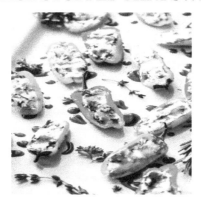

Prep Time: 10mints, Cook Time: 5mints, Total Time: 15mints

Serving: 6

INGREDIENTS

- ➢ 12 ounces mini sweet peppers
- ➢ 4 ounces herbed cheese
- ➢ Alessi's Balsamic Reduction for drizzling

INSTRUCTIONS

- ✓ Preheat the stove to 400°F at that point wash and dry the peppers. Cut every one and a half and wipe out the seeds.
- ✓ Line a treat sheet with material paper, organize the peppers on top and heat them in the stove for five mints. Evacuate and permit to cool for 5-10 mints, until sufficiently cool to deal with.

- ✓ Spoon herbed cheddar within each pepper at that point shower with balsamic decrease. Serve quickly or refrigerate for as long as 1 day before serving

CURRY ROASTED VEGETABLE QUINOA BOWLS

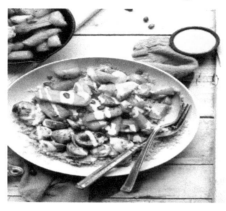

Prep Time: 10mints, Cook Time: 30mints, Total Time: 40mints

Servings: 4

INGREDIENTS

- 1 cup quinoa
- 2 cups vegetable broth
- 1 small head cauliflower
- 1 medium sweet potato
- 1 15oz can chickpeas
- 4 tablespoons olive oil
- 1 teaspoon curry powder
- 1/2 teaspoon turmeric
- 1/2 teaspoon cumin
- 1/2 teaspoon sea salt
- 1/4 teaspoon smoked paprika
- 1 bunch curly kale
- 1 lemon
- Lemon Herb Tahini Dressing or Vegan Ranch

✓ Preheat the range to 425°F. Shower a heating sheet with a non-stick cooking splash. Spot cauliflower, sweet potatoes, and chickpeas at the heating sheet.

✓ In a bit bowl, whisk together three tablespoons olive oil, curry powder, turmeric, cumin, salt, and paprika. Pour dressing over the veggies and toss to consolidate. Cook at the inside tune for 20 - 30 mints, flipping a part of the manner through.

✓ While the greens are boiling, add quinoa and vegetable juices to a touch pan. Heat to the factor of boiling, cowl and decrease to stew for 15 mints. Remove from warmth and allow to chill till organized to serve.

✓ For the kale, begin by removeling the stems, at that factor attack little portions and add it to a large mixing bowl. Shower with an superb tablespoon of olive oil and the juice of the lemon. Back rub together with your palms until the kale has comfy.

✓ At the factor while veggies are completed broiling, remove them from the range and partition between four dishes. Include equal measures of quinoa and kale to the whole thing of the dishes, at that point sprinkle with tahini dressing of selection.

SIMPLE STIR FRY VEGETABLES

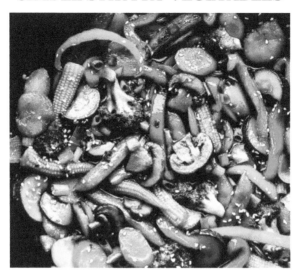

Prep Time: 10mints, Cook time: 15mints, Total time: 25mints

Serving: 4

INGREDIENTS

- 1 cup red onion
- 1 tbsp fresh ginger
- 2 cloves of garlic
- 1 tbsp coconut oil
- 1 green bell pepper
- 1 yellow bell pepper
- 1 red bell pepper
- 2 cups chopped broccoli
- 1 cup button mushrooms
- ½ cup chopped zucchini

INSTRUCTIONS

✓ In an enormous wok soften the coconut oil before including the onion, garlic, and ginger. Sautee delicately on medium warmth until fragrant

✓ Include the remainder of your crude veggies and mix well to cover. Enable the vegetables to cook while mixing for around 5 mints now, you can include a sprinkle of water, cover and permit to cook down until vegetables are cooked yet at the same time crunchy about an extra 10 mints. Include soy sauce or seasonings if utilizing and mix to join before removing the warmth.

VEGAN ASIAN-INSPIRED MEAL PREP BOWL

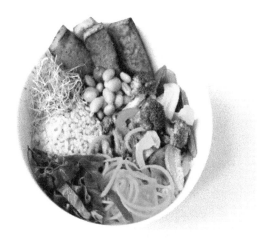

Prep Time: 10mints, Cook time: 10mints, Total time: 20mints

Serving: 4

INGREDIENTS

- 4 servings of Orange Sesame Ginger Tofu
- 4 servings of Simple Stir Fry Vegetables
- 2 cups baby spinach
- 1 cup of boiled and shelled edamame
- 3 carrots
- 1½ cups shredded red cabbage
- 1 cup Alfalfa sprouts
- 2 cups cooked brown rice

✓ Presently comes the fun part - gathering! Set out 4 holders and beginning with the new vegetables, layer with ½ a cup of infant spinach, a bunch of carrots, red cabbage.

✓ Next include ½ a cup of dark colored rice, ¼ cup edamame, and your pan-seared vegetables. Top with your heated tofu and horse feed grows

ROASTED CHICKPEA TRAIL MIX

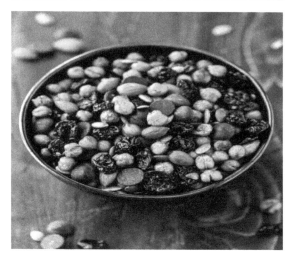

Prep Time: 5mints, Total Time: 10mints

Servings: 1 /4 cup

INGREDIENTS

- 2- cups roasted chickpeas
- 1- cup cashews
- ½- cup dried cranberries
- ¼- cup chocolate chips
- ½- cup dried tart cherries
- ¼- cup sunflower seeds
- ½- cup puffed brown rice
- ½- cup dried apricots

✓ Totally cool broiled chickpeas.

✓ Combine all INGREDIENTS: in a huge bowl.

✓ Separate into singular compartments or resealable sacks containing 1/4 cup each.

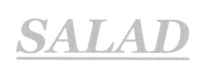

SALAD

THAI CHICKPEA MASON JAR SALAD

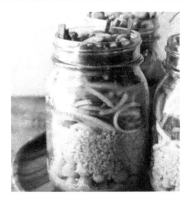

Prep Time: 20mints, Cook Time: 20mints, Total Time: 40mints

Serving: 4

- Jar Salads:
- 3/4 cup uncooked quinoa
- 2 cups chickpeas
- 1 medium-sized zucchini
- 1/2 jumbo carrot
- 1 1/2 cups cabbage
- 1/4 cup honey-roasted peanuts
- Tangy Peanut Dressing:
- 1 tablespoon sesame oil
- 5 tablespoons rice vinegar
- 3 tablespoons peanut butter
- 1 tablespoon maple syrup
- 1 1/2 tablespoons soy sauce
- 1 teaspoon ground ginger

✓ Cook quinoa as per bundle bearings. Put aside to cool.

✓ Shake together dressing INGREDIENTS: and split between 4 1-16 ounces containers, approximately 2 tablespoons for every container.

✓ Include the accompanying request: chickpeas, cooled quinoa, carrot noodles, zucchini noodles, shredded cabbage, nectar simmered peanuts.

✓ Seal and store in the ice chest for as long as 4 days.

✓ To serve, shake everything out into an enormous bowl and enjoy cold.

SOUTHWESTERN SWEET POTATO & LENTIL JAR SALADS

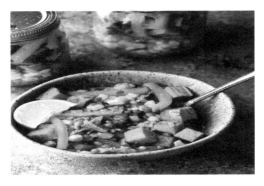

Prep Time: 15mints, Cook Time: 25mints, Total Time: 40mints

Servings: 4

INGREDIENTS

- Chili Lime Vinaigrette
- 2 tablespoons olive oil
- 2 tablespoons white wine vinegar
- 2 teaspoons lime juice
- 1/4 teaspoon salt
- 1/2 teaspoon chili powder
- 1 clove garlic

- 2 teaspoons honey
- Salad
- 6 cups sweet potato cubes
- 1 tablespoon olive oil
- 1/2 teaspoon chili powder
- 19 oz brown lentils
- 11.5- oz corn kernels1 red bell pepper

- ✓ Shake together with or without vinaigrette INGREDIENTS: and set.

- ✓ Warmth the broiler to 425°F. Toss the sweet potato solid shapes in the olive oil and bean stew powder and meal in the stove for 10 mints, turn, at that point prepare for an additional 15 mints or until cooked through.

- ✓ Amass the artisan jolts in the accompanying request:- 1 tablespoon of vinaigrette

- ✓ ½ cup lentils

- ✓ ½ cup corn kernels

- ✓ 1 cup sweet potato cubes

- ✓ bell pepper slices

ROASTED SWEET POTATO & BLACK BEAN SALAD

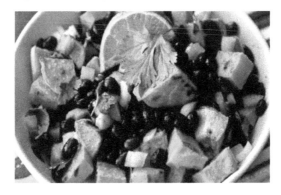

Prep Time: 10mints, Total Time: 10mints

Serving: 3

INGREDIENTS

- ➢ 3 tablespoons Creamy Vegan Avocado Dressing
- ➢ 1/3 cup roasted sweet potato cubes
- ➢ 1/4 cup seasoned black beans
- ➢ 1/4 cup purple cabbage
- ➢ 1/3 cup cooked quinoa
- ➢ 2 cups mixed salad greens

INSTRUCTIONS

- ✓ Layer the INGREDIENTS: in a mason container once cooled and place in the ice chest as follows from base to top
- ✓ Blended Salad Greens Last

✓ In the event that you need to warm a portion of the layers, just separate them on a plate and warm independently.
✓ Enjoy!

FRESH AND EASY GREEN LENTIL SALAD RECIPE

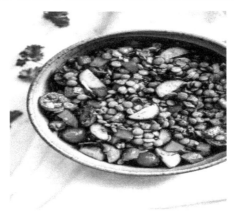

Prep Time: 10mints, Cook Time: 30mints, Total Time: 40mints

Servings: 4

INGREDIENTS

- 3/4 cup uncooked green lentils
- 2 cups of water
- 1 red bell pepper
- 2 Persian cucumbers
- Large handful little tomatoes
- 1 tablespoon capers
- 2 tablespoons red onion
- 2 tablespoons fresh parsley
- 1 tablespoon fresh mints
- Juice of 1/2 lemon
- 1 tablespoon olive oil
- Salt & pepper

✓ Rince the lentils and add them to a medium pot alongside the two cups of water over medium-excessive warm temperatures.

✓ Return to a fast stew at that point lessen the hot heat so it tenderly stews for 30-40mints or till the lentils are cooked.

✓ In the imply time, prep exceptional INGREDIENTS: and add them to a medium serving of mixed greens bowl.

✓ At the point, while the lentils are finished, channel them and rince with cool water and afterward channel them once more and add them to the serving of blended greens bowl.

✓ Include the lemon juice and olive oil. Add salt and pepper to flavor.

✓ Serving of combined greens will keep for a couple of days in the ice chest.

MOROCCAN QUINOA, CARROT, AND CHICKPEA SALAD

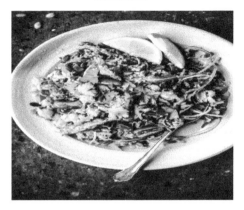

Prep Time: 15mints, Total Time: 15mints

Serving: 4

- 2- cups cooked quinoa
- 1- cup cooked chickpeas
- 1- cup carrots
- ¼- cup dates
- 2- cups rucola or other baby greens
- ¼- cup sunflower seeds
- ¼- cup pepitas, pumpkin seeds
- ½- cup parsley
- 1- clove garlic
- Lemon Ginger Vinaigrette
- ¼- cup olive oil
- Juice of a lemon, ~3 tablespoons
- ½- teaspoon fresh ginger
- ½- teaspoon sea salt
- ½- teaspoon maple syrup or honey

- ➤ ½- teaspoon cinnamon
- ➤ ¼- teaspoon cayenne pepper
- ➤ ¼- teaspoon pepper

INSTRUCTIONS

- ✓ Add the entirety of the INGREDIENTS: to an enormous bowl and top with the vinaigrette. Blend well, until completely joined, and serve.

- ✓ Keep remains in the fridge for two or three days, or longer without the greens blended in. It tends to be served cold or at room temperature and is best in the wake of sitting for in any event 60 mints.

- ✓ To make the vinaigrette, add the entirety of the INGREDIENTS: to a container or little bowl and blend until joined.

VEGAN CHOPPED SALAD WITH SPICED CHICKPEAS

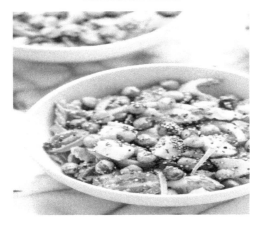

Prep Time: 10mints, Total Time: 10mints

Servings: 4

- for the dressing:
- 3 tablespoons tahini
- 2 tablespoons fresh lemon juice
- 1 garlic clove
- 1 - 2 tablespoons
- Pinch of salt
- for the salad:
- 2 romaine hearts
- 1 medium cucumber
- 1-pint grape tomatoes halved
- 1/3 cup chopped pitted kalamata olives
- 1/2 cup red onion
- 1 batch spiced chickpeas + quinoa

INSTRUCTIONS

- ✓ For the dressing, in a little bowl, whisk together the tahini, lemon juice and 2 tablespoons of water. Race in garlic, tarragon, and salt.

- ✓ For the serving of mixed greens, in an enormous bowl, toss together the romaine, cucumber, tomatoes, olives, and onion. Add dressing and toss to cover.

- ✓ Serve into bowls and top with heartily spiced chickpeas.

CHICKPEA & QUINOA MASON JAR SALAD

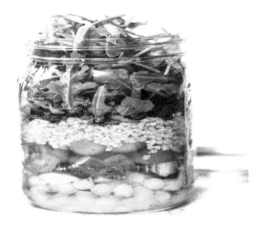

Prep Time: 5mints, Total Time: 5mints

Servings: 2

INGREDIENTS

- for the salad:
- 1 cup canned chickpeas
- 1 cup chopped cucumbers
- 1 cup chopped cherry tomatoes
- 1 cup cooked quinoa
- 1/2 cup chopped flat-leaf parsley
- 3 - 4 cups arugula

- For the dressing:
- 2 tablespoon olive oil
- Juice of 1 lemon
- 1 teaspoon dijon mustard
- 1 teaspoon maple syrup
- 1/2 teaspoon garlic powder
- Salt & pepper

✓ Start with the dressing. Whisk all INGREDIENTS: together in a little bowl. Taste and modify flavoring whenever wanted.

✓ At the point when prepared to amass the servings of mixed greens, equitably isolate the dressing between 2 wide-mouth artisan containers.

✓ At that point equitably separate the rest of the INGREDIENTS: and add to the artisan shakes in the request recorded. Seal with top and store in the cooler until prepared to eat.

✓ When serving, pour the substance of the mason container into a bowl. Mix around to help get dressing dispersed and enjoy!

SMOOTHIES

MEAL PREP STRAWBERRY BANANA SPINACH SMOOTHIE

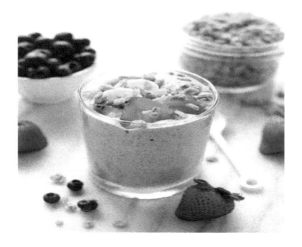

Prep Time: 5mints, Total Time: 5mints

Serving: 4

INGREDIENTS

- For the Meal Prep Smoothies Bags
- 2 cups frozen sliced bananas
- 2 cups frozen whole strawberries
- 4 cups fresh spinach
- 4 teaspoons chia seeds
- For Serving
- 2 tablespoons vanilla protein powder
- 1/2 cup unsweetened almond milk

INSTRUCTIONS

✓ **For the Bag:** In the first place, line a heating sheet with material paper. At that point, uniformly spread out 2 cups of cut bananas, 2 cups of entire strawberries. Spot in the cooler for around 2 hours or until totally solidified.

✓ Next, take 4 quart-size cooler sacks and compose the date and Strawberry Banana Green Smoothie on the front. Include 1 cup of the solidified organic product, a bunch of spinach, and a teaspoon of chia seeds to each pack.

✓ Prior to ingredient, ensure you press however much let some circulation into as could be expected to forestall cooler consume. Seal and spot in the cooler for later use.

✓ **For Blending:** When you're prepared to mix, the void substance of spinach smoothie sack into a rapid blender

✓ At that point, include around 1/2 cup of almond milk and 2 tablespoons of your preferred protein powder.

✓ Mix on high for around 1 moment or until everything is mixed

BERRY SMOOTHIE BOWLS

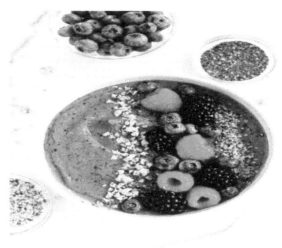

Prep Time: 10mints, Total Time: 10mints

Serving: 2

INGREDIENTS

- 1- Frozen Banana,
- 1- Tablespoon Almond Butter,
- 2/3- cup Almond Milk,
- 1- cup Fresh Raspberries.
- Suggested Toppings:
- Fresh Raspberries
- Chia Seeds
- Fresh Blueberries
- Shredded Coconut
- Banana
- Mints Leaves
- Dark Chocolate
- Mixed nuts and seeds

✓ Find all INGREDIENTS: in a blender and mix for 30 seconds or till completely creamy. Top as desired and serve.

TROPICAL SMOOTHIE BOWLS

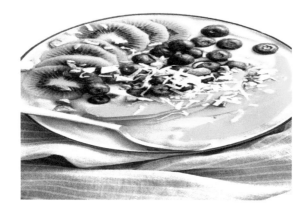

Prep Time: 10mints, Total Time: 10mints

Serving: 1

INGREDIENTS

- 1 Frozen Banana
- 1 Tablespoon Almond Butter
- 2/3 cup Almond Milk
- 1/2 a Fresh Mango
- 1/2 a Fresh Papaya
- Suggested Toppings:
- Chia Seeds
- Fresh Blueberries
- Shredded Coconut
- Mints Leaves
- Fresh chopped Mango
- Mixed nuts and seeds

✓ Put all INGREDIENTS: in a blender and join for 30 seconds or until splendidly scrumptious. Top as needed and serve.

GREEN SMOOTHIE BOWLS

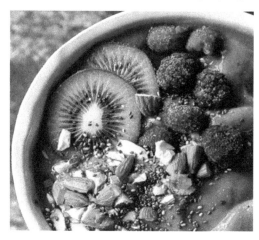

Prep Time: 5mints, Total Time: 5mints

Serves 1

INGREDIENTS

- 1 Frozen Banana
- 1 Tablespoon Almond Butter
- 2/3 cup Almond Milk
- Large Handful Fresh Baby Spinach
- 1 Apple
- A squeeze of lime juice

- Suggested Toppings:
- Fresh Raspberries
- Chia Seeds
- Fresh Blueberries
- Shredded Coconut
- Banana
- Mixed nuts and seeds

✓ Locate all INGREDIENTS: in a blender and blend for 30 seconds or till entirely stable. Top as required and serve.

CREAMY AVOCADO BANANA GREEN SMOOTHIE

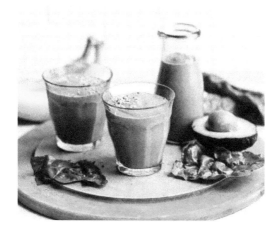

Prep Time: 5mints, Total Time: 5mints

Servings: 2

- ➢ SMOOTHIE
- ➢ 1- large frozen banana
- ➢ ¼ – ½ - medium ripe avocado
- ➢ 1- scoop plain or vanilla protein powder
- ➢ 1- large handful greens of choice
- ➢ ¾ – 1 cup unsweetened plain almond milk
- ➢ ADD-INS optional
- ➢ 1- Tbsp seed of choice
- ➢ ½- tsp adaptogen of choice
- ➢ ½- cup sliced frozen cucumber or berries

191

INSTRUCTIONS

- ✓ To a fast blender, include solidified banana, avocado, protein powder of decision, greens, and sans dairy milk. As of now, include any ideal include ins, for example, adaptogens, seeds, or extra leafy foods.

- ✓ Mix on high until rich and smooth, scratching drawbacks varying. In the event that the smoothie is excessively thick, add more sans dairy milk to thin. In the event that excessively meager, include increasingly solidified banana or avocado.

- ✓ Taste and change enhance varying, including more banana for sweetness, avocado for smoothness, or greens for dynamic green shading. Protein powder can likewise be utilized to include more sweetness.

- ✓ The partition between serving glasses and enjoy! Best when new, however, scraps will keep concealed in the fridge to 24 hours or in the cooler as long as about fourteen days.

CHOCOLATE ALMOND BUTTER SMOOTHIE BOWL

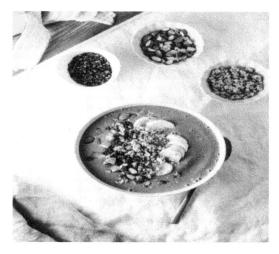

Prep Time: 5mints, Total Time: 5mints

Serving: 2

INGREDIENTS

- 2 large frozen bananas
- 1/4 cup almond butter
- 2 tablespoons cocoa powder
- 1/2 teaspoon vanilla extract
- 1 cup unsweetened almond milk
- 3 – 4 ice cubes
- Optional toppings:
- Bananas
- granola
- cocoa nibs
- chopped almonds

✓ Spot bananas, almond spread, cocoa powder, discretionary vanilla, milk, and ice 3D shapes into the blender, mix until smooth.

✓ Serve in little to medium-sized dishes with discretionary INGREDIENTS: of decision. For an increasingly customary smoothie, serve in a glass with a couple of the discretionary INGREDIENTS:. Utilize a wide straw or spoon.

ORANGE SESAME GINGER TOFU

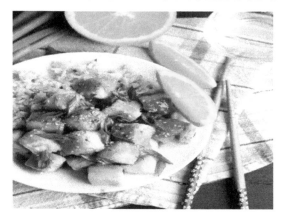

Prep Time: 10mints, Cook time: 25mints, Total time: 35mints

Serving: 7

INGREDIENTS

- 1 20 oz container of extra firm tofu
- Juice of half an orange
- Juice of one lemon
- 1 tbsp rice wine vinegar
- 1 tbsp freshly grated ginger
- 3 cloves of garlic
- 2 tbsp Bragg's liquid aminos
- 1 tbsp toasted sesame oil
- Black pepper
- ½-1/3 cup warm water

INSTRUCTIONS

✓ Remove the tofu from the bundling and channel the water well, squeezing it with paper towels tenderly to ingest a few overabundance dampness. Cut it up into equal square shapes and break up through what number of servings you are making. A 20 ozpackage should yield 7 servings, so you could have extra more however the marinade is sufficient for the complete institution.

✓ Add the marinade INGREDIENTS: to a little bowl and whisk properly to join - taste to modify flavorings various.

✓ Layer your tofu cuts in a shallow Tupperware field and pour the marinade on top. Permit to marinate inside the ice chest for 60 mints, flipping the case within the center of to assure equivalent flavor assimilation all around.

✓ When carried out, preheat your broiler to 190 C.

✓ Collect the tofu in a heating dish and drench any residual marinade on top. Spread the dish with thwart and put together for 20 mints earlier than flipping and cooking for a further 15 mints revealed.

- ✓ On the off threat that you have an air-fryer, you can cook them at one hundred seventy for round 12-15 mints, sincerely do not empty any overabundance marinade into the crate

TROPICAL GREEN

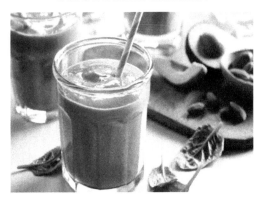

Prep Time: 5mints, Total time: 15mints

Serving: 2

- ➢ 1- cup fresh mango
- ➢ 1- cup fresh pineapple
- ➢ 3- tablespoons hemp seeds
- ➢ 2- cups baby kale/spinach
- ➢ 1 ½- cups Almond Breeze Unsweetened Vanilla Almond Coconut Blend

- ✓ Include the natural product, hemp seeds, and greens into a little pack and spot in the cooler.

- ✓ At the point when prepared to mix, include smoothie pack, alongside the almond milk, and mix until smooth.

CHOCOLATE STRAWBERRY

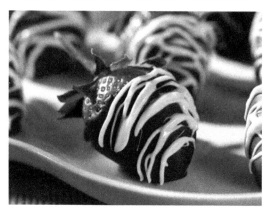

Prep Time: 5mints, Total time: 15mints

Serving: 2

INGREDIENTS

- ➤ 1- medium banana
- ➤ 2- cups fresh strawberries
- ➤ 1 ½- cups Almond Breeze Unsweetened Chocolate Almond milk

INSTRUCTIONS

- ✓ Include the organic product into a little pack and spot it in the cooler.

- ✓ At the point when prepared to mix, include the smoothie pack, alongside the almond milk, and mix until smooth.

RASPBERRY DARK CHOCOLATE OVERNIGHT QUINOA

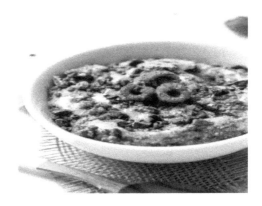

Prep Time: 5mints, Total Time: 1hr 5mints

Servings: 2

INGREDIENTS

- 1/3- cup quinoa flakes
- 1/3- cup cooked quinoa
- 2- tablespoons chia seeds
- 1- tablespoon raw cacao powder
- 1- tablespoon chocolate protein powder
- 1- tablespoon chocolate green powder
- 1 ½- cups non-dairy milk
- 1- tablespoon maple syrup
- ¼- cup raspberries
- Cacao nibs to garnish
- Almond butter

- ✓ Add all INGREDIENTS: to an enormous artisan container or fixed compartment. Mix until completely fused and everything looks decent and chocolate.

- ✓ Fix the top and spot in the cooler to sit medium-term

- ✓ Remove and move to a bowl and enhancement with cleaved almonds. Enjoy

GINGERBREAD GRANOLA

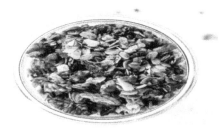

Prep Time: 10mints, Cook Time: 30mints, Total Time: 40mints

Serving: 8 cups

- 4 cups old-fashioned rolled oats
- 1 ½ cups raw pecans and/or walnuts
- 1 teaspoon fine-grain sea salt
- 1 teaspoon ground cinnamon
- 1 teaspoon ground ginger
- ½ cup melted coconut oil
- ⅓ cup real maple syrup
- ¼ cup molasses
- 1 teaspoon vanilla extract
- ½ cup large, unsweetened coconut flakes
- ⅓ cup chopped dried cranberries
- ⅓ cup chopped candied ginger

- ✓ Preheat the broiler to 350 levels Fahrenheit and line a half of-sheet field with cloth paper. In a massive blending bowl, consolidate the oats, nuts, salt, cinnamon, and ground ginger. Mix to consolidate.

- ✓ Mix within the oil, maple syrup, molasses, and vanilla. Turn the granola out onto your readied skillet and make use of an vast spoon to unfold it in an even layer. Heat for 10 mints, at that factor, remove from the broiler and top with coconut portions. Work up the combination to make certain the granola chefs similarly.

- ✓ Return the container to the broiler for eight to 11 additional mints, or until the granola is softly fantastic on pinnacle. It will preserve on crisping up because it cools.

- ✓ Top the granola with the cleaved cranberries and sugar-coated ginger. Let the granola cool earlier than breaking it into portions and getting a rate out of it.

- ✓ Store the granola in a hermetically sealed holder. It have to remain crisp for 1 to approximately fourteen days. Store in the refrigerator for a extra drawn out time span of usability.

DESSERT

VEGAN NO-BAKE TRAIL MIX GRANOLA BARS

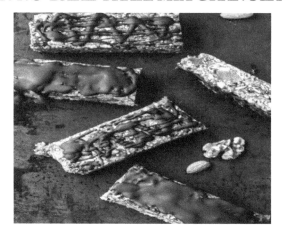

Prep Time: 10mints, Total Time: 10mints

Servings: 10 bars

INGREDIENTS

- 1 ½ cups nuts and seeds of choice
- ½ cup flaked coconut toasted
- ½ cup dried fruit of choice
- 1 tablespoon chia seeds
- ¼ teaspoon kosher salt
- ½ teaspoon cinnamon
- ½ cup creamy almond butter
- ⅓ cup maple syrup
- 2 tablespoons coconut oil
- 1 teaspoon vanilla extract

INSTRUCTIONS

✓ Line an 8x8" square container with material paper and daintily oil with coconut oil. Put in a safe spot.

✓ In an enormous blending bowl, mix together the nuts and seeds, chipped coconut, dried natural product, chia seeds, legitimate salt, and cinnamon.

✓ Mix together the almond margarine, maple syrup, and coconut oil in a little microwave-safe bowl or fluid estimating cup.

✓ Microwave the blend for 30 seconds - it ought to be hot and pour effectively. Mix in the vanilla concentrate.

✓ Pour the almond spread/maple syrup blend over the dry INGREDIENTS: and mix until the entirety of the dry INGREDIENTS: is covered.

✓ Empty the clingy blend into the readied dish and afterward utilize a level bottomed drinking glass, estimating cup, or spatula to press the blend into a firm, even layer in the skillet.

✓ Spread and spot in the fridge for in any event 1 hour before cutting into 10 granola bars - the more you let them sit, the less brittle they'll be the point at which you cut into them.

✓ Store the granola bars in a fixed sack or compartment in the fridge for about fourteen days or in the cooler for a couple of months.

VEGAN RASPBERRY OATMEAL BARS

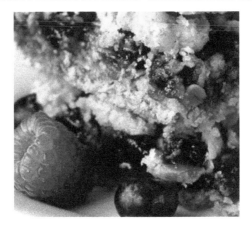

Prep Time: 15mints, Cook Time: 30mints, Total Time: 45mints

Serving: 12

- For the raspberry chia jam:
- 2 cups frozen raspberries
- 2 tbsp chia seeds
- 3 tbsp pure maple syrup
- For the bars:
- 1 cup oat flour
- 1½ cups old-fashioned oats
- 2 tbsp coconut sugar
- ½ tsp cinnamon
- ¼ tsp fine sea salt
- ½ tsp baking soda
- ½ cup unsweetened applesauce
- ¼ cup pure maple syrup
- ¼ cup coconut oil
- 1/2 tsp vanilla extract
- 1/2 tsp almond extract

INSTRUCTIONS

- ✓ Preheat stove to 325F. Oil an 8x8in heating dish with coconut oil or cooking shower.

- ✓ Warmth a little pot over medium warmth. Include raspberries, chia seeds, and maple syrup. Cook for around 8-10 mints, blending regularly. Utilize a potato masher to crush berries for the "jam" layer. Put aside to cool

- ✓ Consolidate oats, oat flour, sugar, cinnamon salt, and heating soft drink in an enormous bowl.

- ✓ Include fruit purée, maple syrup and coconut oil, vanilla, and almond remove, blending to join.

- ✓ Put aside a storing half cup of the oat blend and afterward spoon the rest equally into the readied container. Top with raspberry chia jam, spreading uniformly with a spoon or spatula.

- ✓ Drop the remainder of the oat blend on top.

- ✓ Heat for 30 mints. Cool totally on a wire rack before cutting into 12 bars. Store bars in a sealed shut compartment in the cooler.

VEGAN NO-BAKE PISTACHIO COOKIES RECIPE

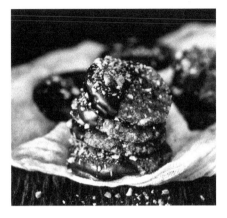

Prep Time: 5mints, Cooking Time: 10mints, Total Time: 15mints

Serving: 16 cookies

INGREDIENTS

- ➢ Cookies:
- ➢ 1 cup pistachios
- ➢ 1/2 cup unsweetened shredded coconut
- ➢ 1/4 cup gluten-free rolled oats
- ➢ 2 tbsp maple syrup
- ➢ 1 tbsp moringa powder
- ➢ 1-2 tbsp water
- ➢ 1 tsp vanilla extract
- ➢ Filling:
- ➢ 1 cup unsweetened shredded coconut
- ➢ 1/2 cup raw cashews
- ➢ 1/4 cup gluten-free rolled oats
- ➢ 2 tbsp almond butter
- ➢ 1 tsp vanilla
- ➢ 1 tbsp coconut oil

✓ Spot the treat INGREDIENTS: in your nourishment processor and heartbeat until joined or until the blend meets up.

✓ Spot the blend between two bits of cling wrap, and utilize a moving pin to roll the treat batter until it gets around 1/2 inch thick. With a round cutout, cut treats out until you have no more mixture. Set the treats in the cooler for 5-10 mints to solidify.

✓ Meanwhile, set up the filling by setting the INGREDIENTS: in the nourishment processor and beating the blend until it is pleasant and smooth.

✓ Remove the treats from the cooler and scoop around 1-2 tablespoons of the filling over a portion of the treats. Spot another treat over the filling to amass the treat sandwiches.

✓ Enjoy promptly or store treats in the cooler for as long as multi-week.

BLUEBERRY OAT FLOUR WAFFLES

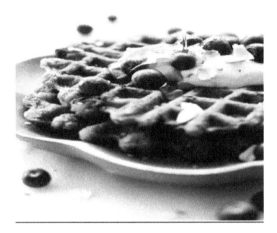

Prep Time: 5mints, Cook Time: 6mints, Total Time: 11mints

Serving: 2 large waffles

INGREDIENTS

- 1 cup oat flour
- 1 tbsp baking powder
- ½ cup unsweetened applesauce
- ¼ cup non-dairy milk
- 2 tbsp maple syrup
- 1 tsp lemon juice
- ½ tsp vanilla bean powder
- 1/4 cup blueberries
- Toppings: coconut whipped cream

- ✓ Consolidate the entirety other than the blueberries in a fast blender.

- ✓ Mix till very a good deal consolidated, but, don't over blend. You can, then again, integrate eventing by way of flip in a blending bowl.

- ✓ Include the blueberries and heartbeat quick to mixture them in.

- ✓ Splash the waffle iron with coconut oil or nonstick bathe

- ✓ Empty a big part of the hitter right into a preheated waffle iron and prepare dinner as indicated by using manufacturers' INGREDIENTS:

- ✓ Rehash with the rest of the participants.

VANILLA BLUEBERRY CHIA PUDDING

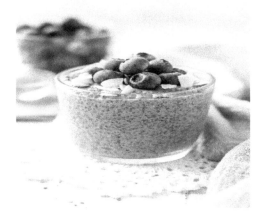

Prep Time: 5mints, Total Time: 5mints

Servings: 2 Glasses

INGREDIENTS

- 4- Tbsp Chia Seeds
- 2- Tbsp Xylitol
- 2- tsp Vanilla Essence
- ¾- Cup Almond Milk or Oat Milk or any form of milk
- ½- Cup Frozen/Fresh Blueberries

INSTRUCTIONS

- ✓ In a little bowl, combine the milk, xylitol, and vanilla.

- ✓ Blend in the Chia Seeds

- ✓ Empty the blend into glasses, including a couple of blueberries midway.

- ✓ Spot in the ice chest medium-term.

- ✓ Top with more blueberries.

- ✓ Enjoy.

BLACK BEAN BAKED TAQUITOS

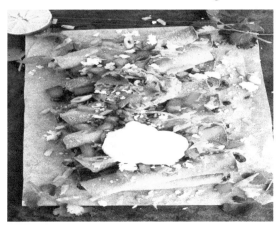

Prep Time: 15mints, Cook Time: 30mints, Total Time: 45mints

Servings: 10 taquitos

INGREDIENTS

- 6 cups sweet potato cubes
- juice of 1 lime
- 1 1/2 tablespoons fajita seasoning
- 1 cup black beans
- 1 1/2 cups shredded cheese optional

- 10 tortillas
- spray oil
- Suggested toppings:
- guacamole
- yogurt
- pico de gallo
- cilantro

- ✓ Fill a common-sized container with 2 cups of water and find a steamer crate on the cover.

- ✓ Arrange sweet potato stable shapes on the steamer bushel.

- ✓ Steam for 20-half-hour, till the sweet potatoes, are fork-sensitive.

- ✓ Include the lime juice and fajita flavoring, and pound till wealthy and smooth.

- ✓ Foll within the cheddar and dark beans.

- ✓ Roll taquitos: region 1/four - 1/3 cup of filling on an eight-inch tortilla.

- ✓ Move firmly and area crease side down in a nine x 13-inch dish or on a heating sheet. Rehash, settling the rest of the taquitos in firmly.

- ✓ Splash with oil anywhere.

- ✓ Prepare for 7-15 mints, till darkish-colored and fresh.

CHOCOLATE PEANUT BUTTER CHIA PUDDING

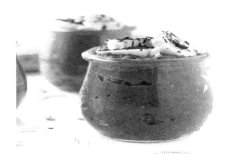

Prep Time: 20mints, Total Time: 20mints

Servings: 4

INGREDIENTS

- For the peanut butter layer:
- 1- cup almond milk
- 3- tablespoons peanut butter
- 1-2- tablespoons maple syrup
- ¼- cup chia seeds
- ⅛- teaspoon kosher salt
- For the chocolate layer:

- 1- cup almond milk
- 2- tablespoons cocoa powder
- 1- tablespoon peanut butter
- 2-3- tablespoons maple syrup
- ¼- cup chia seeds
- ⅛- teaspoon kosher salt

INSTRUCTIONS

- ✓ In a bowl or fluid estimating cup, whisk together the entirety of the INGREDIENTS: in the nutty spread layer. Let gel for around 10 mints, and afterward, move to a blender. Mix until smooth. Remove from blender into a bowl or fluid estimating cup and put it in a safe spot. Rehash steps to make the chocolate layer, no compelling reason to wash the blender between layers.

- ✓ When the two layers are made, layer the chocolate and nutty spread puddings in little containers or cups, substituting as wanted. Refrigerate for at any rate 2 hours before serving.

- ✓ On the other hand, on the off chance that you don't need the chia pudding mixed, mix together the elements for the nutty spread layer in one bowl, and mix together the elements for the chocolate layer in another.

- ✓ Let them each set for in any event 2 hours in the fridge, and afterward layered into cups or containers.

- ✓ Store in the cooler. Top with a shower of nutty spread and a sprinkle of chocolate chips or cacao nibs to serve!

BASIC HOUMOUS RECIPE

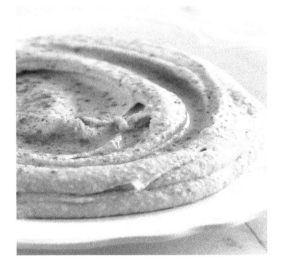

Prep Time: 5mints, Cooking Time: 10mints, Total Time: 15mints

Serving: 6-8

INGREDIENTS

- 400g of chickpeas
- 4- tsp tahini
- 2- garlic cloves
- 1- tsp crushed sea salt
- 6- tbsp quality extra virgin olive oil
- 3½- tbsp freshly squeezed lemon juice
- Paprika
- Coriander or parsley leaves

✓ Wash the chickpeas in chilly water and tip into the nourishment processor.

✓ Include the tahini, squashed garlic, salt, lemon juice and seven tablespoons of the saved fluid from the jars.

✓ Turn on the nourishment processor and gradually pour in the oil while it runs.

✓ At the point when the blend is completely joined and smooth, tip it into a serving dish.

✓ Sprinkle with some progressively additional virgin olive oil and beautify with a couple of entire chickpeas.

✓ Sprinkle with paprika and finely cleaved coriander or parsley leaves, for shading.